Brief Psychosocial Intervention for Adolescents

Brief Psychosocial Intervention for Adolescents

Keep It Simple; Do It Well

Ian Goodyer
University of Cambridge

Raphael Kelvin
National Clinical Lead MindEd
Technology Enhanced Learning
NHS Health Education England

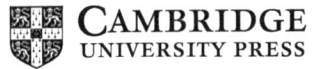

CAMBRIDGE
UNIVERSITY PRESS

CAMBRIDGE
UNIVERSITY PRESS

University Printing House, Cambridge CB2 8BS, United Kingdom

One Liberty Plaza, 20th Floor, New York, NY 10006, USA

477 Williamstown Road, Port Melbourne, VIC 3207, Australia

314–321, 3rd Floor, Plot 3, Splendor Forum, Jasola District Centre, New Delhi – 110025, India

103 Penang Road, #05–06/07, Visioncrest Commercial, Singapore 238467

Cambridge University Press is part of the University of Cambridge.

It furthers the University's mission by disseminating knowledge in the pursuit of education, learning, and research at the highest international levels of excellence.

www.cambridge.org
Information on this title: www.cambridge.org/9781108984546
DOI: 10.1017/9781108989442

First published 2023

A catalogue record for this publication is available from the British Library.

Library of Congress Cataloging-in-Publication Data
Names: Goodyer, Ian M., author. | Kelvin, Raphael, author.
Title: Brief psychosocial intervention for adolescents : keep it simple ; do it well / Ian Goodyer, University of Cambridge, Raphael Kelvin, MindEd, UK.
Description: Cambridge, United Kingdom ; New York, NY : Cambridge University Press, 2022. | Includes index.
Identifiers: LCCN 2022016953 (print) | LCCN 2022016954 (ebook) | ISBN 9781108984546 (paperback) | ISBN 9781108989442 (ebook)
Subjects: LCSH: Brief psychotherapy for teenagers. | Adolescent psychotherapy. | BISAC: PSYCHOLOGY / Mental Health
Classification: LCC RJ504.3 .G66 2022 (print) | LCC RJ504.3 (ebook) | DDC 616.89/140835–dc23/eng/20220629
LC record available at https://lccn.loc.gov/2022016953
LC ebook record available at https://lccn.loc.gov/2022016954

ISBN 978-1-108-98454-6 Paperback

Contents

Acknowledgements

We recognise and thank the many clinical scientists, mental health practitioners, therapists and health care managers who made the writing of this book possible. In particular, we thank Professor Bernadka Dubicka of the Hull York Medical School and Professor Paul Wilkinson of the University of Cambridge, who contributed substantially to the development, clinical research and evaluation of brief psychosocial intervention (BPI). The clinical science that has established BPI as clinically effective for the treatment of major depression in adolescents was funded by the National Institute of Health and Care Research UK, together with supporting funds from the Wellcome Trust, Medical Research Council (MRC) UK and the universities of Cambridge, Manchester, Reading and University College London. We are grateful to the National Institute for Health and Care Excellence (NICE) UK for adopting and recognising BPI as an evidence-based clinical intervention for the treatment of major depression in adolescents. We pay tribute to the NHS organisations who sponsored the randomised controlled trials to ensure that BPI was tested against proven psychotherapies, thereby ensuring the best pragmatic results for the benefit of mentally unwell young people. Finally, we thank all the young people, parents and carers who helped and participated in our studies and who received treatment in our clinics throughout the NHS in England. Their lived experiences of mental illness and their perception of BPI treatment have made an invaluable contribution to our understanding of therapeutic effects. We sincerely hope that in return this book contributes to future improvements in the treatment and care of young people with depression and related mental illnesses and their families through the delivery of evidence-based psychosocial interventions such as BPI.

1   Adolescence and the Psychotherapies

Adolescence and Mental Health

The notion that the teenage years have any particular value in social, cultural or biological terms does not appear in any literature until the fifteenth century. Before then, received wisdom was that infancy and childhood were followed by adulthood and all that goes with being a grown-up individual in any society. The word 'adolescence' came from the Latin word *adolescere*, meaning 'to grow up or to grow into maturity'. Although ongoing maturation during the teenage years is clearly suggested, there appears to be no formal adoption of the concept in any society until the early twentieth century. In 1904 the first president of the American Psychological Association, Greville Stanley Hall, was credited with coining the term 'adolescence'. In his study entitled *Adolescence*, he described this new developmental phase, which he hypothesised came about due to social changes. Some of this hypothesis resonates clearly with today's viewpoints, although much is also now known to be incorrect. Hall considered that the evidence supporting a rise in depressed mood during the adolescent years stemmed from being disliked by peers and interpersonal adversity influencing social-affective development such as the formation of negative memories. Hall also noted the emergence of delinquency and listed risk factors markedly similar to those reported by today's behavioural scientists, such as family-centred childhood adversities. Finally, Hall observed that adolescents had a heightened sense of sensation-seeking, risk-taking and sensitivity to the media. Hall drew on an immense amount of pre-existing knowledge, making it clear that much was already known about the adolescent period of the life-course. Perhaps Hall's achievement was to draw together existing knowledge into one place and add many insights of his own. From the practice perspective, the development of adolescent-specific social policy, education and medicine can in part be attributed to this period of the early twentieth century. The creation of high schools, correctional centres and medical services that focused on the particular needs of adolescents stems from Hall and subsequent scholars, policy-makers and practitioners of the early twentieth century.

Today the World Health Organization (WHO) recognises adolescence as a crucial period in the development of a human being. The WHO recently noted the following key facts about the adolescent years, shown in Table 1.1. Over the 100 years since Hall's seminal work and coining of the term, the WHO (the organisation that sets the agenda for health for governments worldwide) considers the mental health of adolescents aged 10 to 19 years one of the key agendas for the twenty-first century. The WHO has stated that it is crucial to address the needs of adolescents with defined mental health conditions. A suggested set of policy principles for practice is: avoiding institutionalisation and over-medicalisation, prioritising non-pharmacological approaches and respecting the rights of children in line with the United Nations Convention on the Rights of the Child and other human rights. These policy statements and documents are key for upholding the needs of adolescents, including in mental health services. Hall's seminal work establishes some key principles for practice, including a focus on the family environment for adaptive human development through the adolescent as well as childhood years, the critical role of peer group relationships in ongoing social-affective development and the social sensitivities that emerge in the second decade of life, which have a high impact on self-perception and personal competence. Some selected key facts regarding adolescents are shown in Table 1.1.

Table 1.1 Some key facts on adolescence

- One in six people is aged 10–19 years.
- Mental health conditions account for 16% of the global burden of disease and injury in people aged 10–19 years.
- Half of all mental health conditions start by 14 years of age but most cases are undetected and untreated.
- Globally, depression is one of the leading causes of illness and disability among adolescents.
- Suicide is the third leading cause of death in 15–19-year-olds.
- The consequences of not addressing adolescent mental health conditions extend into adulthood, impairing both physical and mental health and limiting opportunities to lead fulfilling lives as adults.

Source: WHO, 'Adolescent mental health', 17 November 2021, www.who.int/news-room/fact-sheets/detail/adolescent-mental-health

The WHO suggests a set of behavioural targets to achieve their proposed goals, shown in Table 1.2.

Table 1.2 WHO behavioural targets to aid health over adolescence

- Adopting healthy sleep patterns.
- Taking regular exercise.
- Developing coping, problem-solving and interpersonal skills.
- Learning to manage emotions.
- Encouraging supportive environments in the family and at school.
- Ensuring a safe and adaptive environment in the wider community.

Determining how to achieve these targets is a work in progress but both a focus on adolescent-sensitive mental health, education and social care policies and an evidence-based methodology for interventions are required at a level well beyond those in use. For example, currently there is very little evidence base to aid decision-making on what works for adolescents with mental health needs. Given an estimated 10% to 20% of adolescents (who make up around 20% of the human population globally) experience mental health conditions. There is an urgent need for interventions that are evidenced and deliverable in community as well as clinical settings. An important context for considering 'talking cures' for adolescent depression and related mental illnesses is our increasing understanding of adolescent development. To date, the majority of psychotherapies are theories and methods developed for adults with mental illness. Some have been modified successfully to be usable for adolescents. In order to appreciate what the best ingredients might be and how these may operate, we begin with a brief introduction to the neurodevelopment features that emerge during the second decade of life.

Adolescent Maturation

Maturing from childhood through to adulthood involves physical changes and transformation in functions that may not be complete until the middle of the third decade of life. The enormous changes in the brain that occur between birth and 35 years of age include substantial reorganisation of the structures and connections of neural circuits with increasing effectiveness in emotional regulation, executive decision-making and behaviour control. Building a mature mind-brain system requires energy, which has to be transported into the nervous system because the brain does not have its own energy stores. Thus, mind-brain building comes at an energy cost and there may be low energy reserves available to fuel defences against emerging mental illnesses, especially in those at a nutritional disadvantage as observed in young people in long-term poverty. Psychological functions associated with maturing neural circuits likely become more reliable and subserve the young person's emerging repertoire of behavioural actions and responses. The WHO notes the value of learning emotion regulation and cognitive controls, together with recommending and promoting an adaptive social environment. As the mind-brain neurometabolic process proceeds, paradoxically so does an increased liability to mental health difficulties. Indeed, the first episodes of common mental illnesses such as depression, psychoses, substance misuse and personality difficulties occur over this period of neuromaturation through the teenage and young adult years.

Here is the dilemma: how does an adolescent with an emerging mental illness transfer resources to reduce mental illness and promote recovery when they are in a high energy demand period in the life-course and energy resources for the brain may be limited? Adolescence is therefore a period of substantial mental health risk to young people at the same time as they are engaged in effective mind-brain building.

This adds a developmental imperative to understanding how to treat and manage the mentally ill adolescent. The implication from neurodevelopment is that early detection and effective treatment of mental illnesses may contribute to protecting normal mind-brain development. Do we have psychosocial interventions for adolescents that are sufficiently effective to treat mental illness and thereby achieve the developmental goal of normal mind-brain building and promoting well-being?

The Talking Cures and Adolescent Mental Health

The notion of a talking cure for mental distress probably developed in the first millennium in the Middle East and Persia (Iran). The West did not really consider psychosocial interventions for mental illness until the advent of moral treatment approaches for 'disturbance of mind' in the eighteenth century. The first strategy was probably one which likely included reasoning, encouragement and group activities – to rehabilitate the 'insane'.

The first professional in Western society to call himself a psychotherapist was Wilhelm Wundt, a professor of physiology who opened the Institute for Experimental Psychology at the University of Leipzig in Germany in 1879. Wundt developed a method of psychological evaluation he termed introspection and took a scientific approach to the study of thoughts, feelings and sensations that was the forerunner of modern cognitive psychology. His work influenced Greville Stanley Hall and also Sigmund Freud. He trained over 100 students in the new field of psychology and they helped spread the introspective method to aid the study of one's own mind, a technique that lasted formally into the 1920s. By the middle of the twentieth century, the influence of Sigmund Freud on psychological thinking and practice had over-taken Wundt's theories.

From the 1920s through to the present era, there has been a marked expansion in talking cures and their assorted theories. A formalising of psychology and psychotherapy education followed, together with the rules and regulations regarding clinical practice. Over the past century, there have been literally thousands of modifications of psychotherapy theory regarding the formation of mental illnesses and the talking methods to treat these. Psychoanalytic methods proposed by Freud diversified between the First World War and the Second World War and codified themselves into schools of psychoanalysis. Behaviourism also emerged in the 1920s and established itself as an effective method of symptom reduction through the application of techniques based on operant and classical conditioning and social learning theory. Two further theories emerged from the 1950s: cognitivism and existential-humanistic therapy. The humanistic movement largely developed from both existential and person-centred psychotherapy, with the work of Dr Carl Rogers being highly influential. Humanistic therapy emphasises the unconscious less and focuses more on promoting positive, holistic change through the development of a supportive, genuine and empathic therapeutic relationship.

Cognitivism emerged in the 1960s through the work of Albert Ellis (rational-emotive-behaviour therapy) and Aaron Beck (cognitive behavioural therapy). Cognitive behavioural therapy (CBT) is oriented towards symptom relief, collaborative empiricism (i.e. therapist and patient working together to establish common goals in treatment) and modifying abnormal core beliefs about the self, the world and the future; this approach has gained widespread acceptance as a primary treatment for numerous disorders and is perhaps the most widely taught and used therapy worldwide. Two further theoretical frameworks emerged from the 1970s: systems theory with an emphasis on interpersonal dynamics between human networks, usually family members, and a return of transpersonal methods with an emphasis on spiritualism and the human experience. In the last 30 to 40 years, there has been a literal explosion of descriptive titles for 'new' psychotherapies, with a current list of over 200 names, most of which are specific outgrowths of the aforementioned ideas but with a particular focus, such as feminist therapy, group therapy and child and adolescent therapy. This expansion has included many publications on how to do therapies of different types with adolescents. Despite this expansion and proliferation of courses and workshops, the current evidence suggests that the outcomes from talking cures for adolescents with mood-related mental illnesses have not changed much in the last three decades and that we are no nearer understanding how the talking cures work or what intervention works best for which patient or condition than we were 30 years ago [1, 2]. Here we consider that, in order to improve psychotherapies for adolescents, we need a scientific approach to evaluation. This is likely to be best achieved through utilising randomised controlled trial (RCT) methodologies which remain sensitive to the importance of the young patient's experience, and investigating how the talking cure reduces mental difficulties. Ideally such RCTs would include investigations of therapeutic mechanisms that reveal how psychotherapies work and what types of disorders or patients respond best.

Science and Psychotherapy

The science of psychotherapy effectiveness is a recent development in talking cures, emerging from the concept of evidence-based medicine (EBM). The principle of EBM is to establish standards, guiding practitioners towards scientifically supported and away from scientifically unsupported interventions. Applying EBM standards to the talking cures is not easy and certainly a 'work in progress'. To date, very few talking cures have met all the required standards in order to be declared a fully evidenced intervention. A full EBM would be achieved if a psychotherapy had shown: studies of acceptable design, sample size, power and statistical inference; an outcome measure independent of symptoms; recording of adverse events and side effects of treatment; and the replication of findings by an independent group. Currently, what constitutes 'good evidence' for psychotherapy effectiveness is a matter of debate [3]. One key element of a talking cure is that it is efficacious – that is, the treatment produces a beneficial effect often measured as a reduction in mental distress and/or personal impairment. Efficacy is, however, frequently sought under conditions that do not exist in the real world and may overestimate the value of a treatment in everyday clinical circumstances. Efficacy can therefore be defined as the performance of an intervention under ideal and fully controlled circumstances. Unfortunately, implementation of a psychotherapy with such proven efficacy in a standard clinical practice may reveal a number of key difficulties in real-world conditions. For example, the precise research treatment procedures may be under-utilised in real-world conditions where clinics are understaffed for the volume of work being undertaken. Indeed, studies of the utilisation of treatments in medicine in general have shown that poor access, level of recommendation, degree of acceptance and adherence rates can lead to interventions considered highly efficacious being less effective in practice than even interventions demonstrated to be less efficacious in ideal research conditions.

In contrast to efficacy, clinical effectiveness refers to the performance of a treatment under 'real-world' conditions. Here a new treatment is compared with an active agent already considered efficacious. The objective is frequently to show that the new treatment is as good (non-inferior) or better (superior) than those in existing practice. Studies undertaken in pragmatic everyday clinical environments have a greater likelihood of accounting for factors in everyday practice that may reduce utilisation and therefore lower the likelihood of a treatment response. Compared with efficacy studies, the patients treated in pragmatic effectiveness studies also tend to be more real-world. For example, efficacy studies frequently seek homogeneous, 'pure' cases of the disorder under investigation with low comorbidities, few concurrent social difficulties and a high probability of adherence to the treatment protocol. In contrast, effectiveness studies enrol patients with heterogeneous clinical presentations referred through the local health care routes with no guarantee of adherence to protocol and an unknown level of additional comorbidities and psychosocial problems. Although efficacy research maximises the likelihood of observing an intervention effect if one exists, effectiveness research accounts for external patient-, provider- and system-level factors that may moderate an intervention's effect. Therefore, effectiveness research can be more relevant for health care decisions by both providers in practice and policy-makers. Differences between efficacy and effectiveness studies are shown in Table 1.3.

Table 1.3 Differences between efficacy and effectiveness studies

	Efficacy study	Effectiveness study
Question	Does the intervention work under ideal circumstances?	Does the intervention work in real-world practice?
Setting	Resource-intensive 'ideal setting'.	Real-world everyday clinical setting.
Study population	Highly selected, homogeneous population. Several exclusion criteria.	Heterogeneous population. Few to no exclusion criteria.
Providers	Highly experienced and trained providers.	Representative usual providers.
Intervention	Strictly enforced and standardised. No concurrent interventions.	Applied with flexibility. Concurrent interventions and cross-over permitted.

In this book we detail a possible theory, practice principles and clinical delivery of brief psychosocial intervention (BPI) for depressed adolescents. The intervention has been developed within an everyday clinical environment from which an evidence base has emerged through two RCTs examining the pragmatic effectiveness of BPI compared with other already evidence-based interventions. The published evidence base has been of sufficient quality for BPI to be adopted by the National Institute of Health and Care Research (NICE) as an approved talking cure treatment for adolescents with depressive illness.

So far we have been describing quantitative research, which is a set of scientific methods for testing a hypothesis based on theory. But what if the adolescent wishes to describe their mental predicament in their own words and provide explanations for how they came to have mental health problems based entirely on their own perceptions of their experience? This subjectivity approach to life events and difficulties is often better revealed by qualitative methods of inquiry, which can be employed scientifically to propose new theoretical possibilities for the clinical effectiveness of a talking cure. The key difference to quantitative methods is that qualitative research does not seek to generalise findings to a wider population. Results from qualitative studies can, however, be hypothesis-forming and can be used in quantitative studies to determine their validity in a selected clinical population receiving a psychotherapy. So a single case study narrative can be a study with results and conclusions in its own right and its conjectures can be formally tested in subsequent populations.

Qualitative research methods aim to describe the subjective thoughts and feelings of study participants, to record participants' experiences of the phenomena of interest such as undergoing a psychotherapy treatment. The common objective is to find explanations for the experiences being recorded in the particular and specific context within which the individual respondent lives. In the context of psychotherapy, qualitative research methods can explore how patients feel about their treatment and about 'being a patient', report their experiences of, say, participating in an RCT or describe the impact of their life circumstances on their mental state. There are many different methods for obtaining qualitative data but one general principle, known as grounded theory, is to undertake data collection to create a theory for future consideration. In psychotherapy research the commonest method used is to interview the respondent about their experiences of treatment and to record the interview. Subsequently, the audio recording is transcribed and the narrative can then be subject to an interrogation for words or phrases that contain specific meanings. This interrogation uses the phenomenology of the narrative to extract themes from phrases or words that describe potentially important concepts whilst undergoing psychotherapy. We describe a selected example of an adolescent who successfully underwent BPI in Chapters 6 and 7. It is important to note that qualitative methods are scientific because they are used within a rigorous methodological framework of data collection, recording, transcription and thematic interrogation. The methods are important for understanding the experience of psychotherapy from the holistic perspective of the adolescent within their particular family, school and personal environments. These methods are quite distinct from case reporting, which provides anecdotes and commentaries on a treatment experience but is unscientific. Such descriptions are not usable as a means to generate theory even at the individual level. Finally, we note the importance of the notion of 'experts by experience', which is defined as involving people (adolescents, for our purposes, and their families) with lived experience of co-producing better mental health care. This gives everyone trying to improve mental health services a far more informed base of knowledge. Qualitative research methods can be applied to experts by experience to extract the themes from their narrative to identify common principles for informing how psychotherapies might work and informing how services can be fashioned to aid clinical effectiveness.

There are now four talking cures that have been approved by NICE as treatments for major depression episodes in adolescents: individual CBT for at least three months should be offered as a first-line psychological treatment; if this treatment is not available or is not considered to meet the needs of the adolescent then a second-line psychotherapy should be considered: this could be IPT-A (interpersonal therapy for adolescents), BPI or psychodynamic psychotherapy. Family therapy (attachment-based or systemic) has also been approved but the evidence for this second-line therapy is the weakest compared with the other three alternatives.

Adolescence and Psychotherapies

Psychotherapy interventions with adolescents were originally based on interventions developed for adults with mental illness. Over the last 60 years, however, practitioners of talking cures with younger people have modified and evolved practice through their clinical experience of treating adolescent patients. With common mental illnesses involving depression, anxiety, self-harm, suicidality, psychoses and drug misuse emerging in the 11 to 19 age range, there is clearly much to be understood about how talking cures exert their effects in the teenage years. A survey of adolescents in the UK in 2020 [4] noted the following key facts about adolescent mental health (Table 1.4), which emphasise the need to develop talking cures that are effective and implementable in clinical and community settings.

Table 1.4 Mental health of young people in England survey, 2020

- One in six (16.0%) children aged 5–16 years were identified as having a probable mental disorder.
- This is an increase from one in nine (10.8%) in 2017.
- The likelihood of a probable mental disorder increased with age.
- The increase was evident in both boys and girls.

The marked increase in adolescents reporting mental health difficulties has led to calls for increases in the adolescent mental health workforce and an expansion of services in communities including schools.

Overall, the general principle that talking cures with adolescents require a set of skills, some of which are specialist to the age range, has gained strong agreement amongst mental health practitioners. Currently, there are considerable numbers of training programmes to provide would-be practitioners with the skills to undertake psychotherapies of different types with adolescents within health care systems worldwide. Some 3 500 anxious and 5 000 depressed adolescents have been enrolled in psychotherapy studies of efficacy and effectiveness over the past 30 years. Overall, the evidence is clear that treatment is efficacious compared with no treatment. Further, most treatments show reasonably equivalent effects for most anxious and depressive conditions. There is, however, an urgent need to improve the precision and the fine-tuning of these treatments to understand how they work and what works best for which patients. Finally, virtually no attention has been paid to the possible harmful effects of psychotherapies that may accrue for some young people. In the subsequent chapters in this book, we describe the evidence that led to the emergence of and evidence for the use of the BPI clinical method. Brief psychosocial intervention offers an alternative therapy for mood-related mental illness that can be practised by mental health staff and provide an additional treatment opportunity for mentally ill adolescents.

REFERENCES

1. Eckshtain D, Kuppens S, Ugueto A, Ng MY, Vaughn-Coaxum R, Corteselli K et al. Meta-analysis: 13-year follow-up of psychotherapy effects on youth depression. *J Am Acad Child Adolesc Psychiatry*. 2020;59(1):45–63.
2. Weisz JR, Kuppens S, Ng MY, Eckshtain D, Ugueto AM, Vaughn-Coaxum R et al. What five decades of research tells us about the effects

of youth psychological therapy: A multilevel meta-analysis and implications for science and practice. *Am Psychol.* 2017;72(2):79–117.

3. Lilienfeld SO. What is 'evidence' in psychotherapies? *World Psychiatry.* 2019;18(3):245–6.

4. NHS Digital. *Mental Health of Children and Young People in England, 2020: Wave 1 Follow up to the 2017 Survey.* London: NHS Digital, UK, 2020.

2   Evidence-Based Psychotherapy

In the previous chapter we outlined a brief history of psychotherapies since the medieval period and noted that we are now in a scientific phase that is particularly focused on establishing valid clinical effects for talking cures.

Evidence-Based Practice

The principles of how to practise psychotherapies from a scientific perspective originated with the emergence of evidence-based medicine (EBM), which we briefly outlined in Chapter 1. Here we provide a little more detail relevant to practice within mental health services and suggest principles for psychotherapy in routine adolescent mental health treatment.

A clinical pioneer of EBM was Archibald Cochrane (1909–88), a Scottish physician and epidemiologist who wrote about the importance of systematic practice following his alarm at the marked inequalities in the care between the rich and the poor. Cochrane also noted that the physician had little knowledge of which accessible drugs and devices were effective. Further, the demand for treatment was always likely to outstrip available resources, encouraging prescribing through patient demand. As well as noting the absence of knowledge regarding the clinical effectiveness of treatments, Cochrane argued 'that cure is rare while the need for care is widespread, and that the pursuit of cure at all costs may restrict the supply of care' [1]. Cochrane's pioneering agenda was rewarded in 1993 by the formation of the Cochrane Collaboration (www.cochrane.org), a worldwide network of more than 28 000 scientists. This amazing collaboration works to determine and bring to the health care practitioner the best evidence for treatment across a wide range of topics. There are over 6 616 online systematic reviews of health interventions, including the psychotherapies, evaluated by RCTs. In addition, the Cochrane Library links to the Cochrane Central Register of Controlled Trials (CENTRAL), a repository of reports on RCTs and quasi-RCTs. Overall, Cochrane's work highlights the value of RCTs, prompting the creation of a centralised resource of expert reviews of trials accessible to practising clinicians and policy-makers. Medicine was not the only profession to recommend an evidence-based approach to clinical practice. Both clinical psychology and social work sought to introduce evidence-based practice principles for their work as long ago as the early twentieth century, indicating the potential influence of scientific principles on social as well as health care [2].

The framework of evidence base introduced by Cochrane was further developed by David Sackett at McMaster University, Canada, and subsequently at the Centre for Evidence Based Medicine at Oxford University [3]. Sackett and colleagues noted that, even when well trained, many physicians paid little attention to the research evidence regarding treatment for the patient's condition, preferring to rely on the teachings, habits and influences they had received from other individuals during their student years. Sackett and colleagues espoused the belief that best practice is achieved through the 'conscientious, explicit, and judicious use of current best evidence in making decisions about the care of individual patients' [3]. The importance of this conjunction cannot be overstated and for mental health practice is the assimilation by the therapist of best evidence (external information) as part of the working collaboration with the individual patient/family and their particular presentation. For BPI and other psychotherapies, this means a therapist integrating individual clinical expertise with the best available external clinical evidence from systematic research and also paying close attention to the experiences and perceptions of therapy from the client's perspective.

By individual clinical expertise we mean the proficiency and judgement that individual clinicians acquire through clinical experience and clinical practice. Increased expertise is reflected in many ways but especially in more effective and efficient assessment and in the more thoughtful identification and compassionate integration of individual patients' predicaments, rights and preferences in making clinical decisions about their care. This means a focus on clinical skill and pragmatic judgements in collaboration with the patient, based on their best interests and not on intuition, guesswork or the word of charismatic others.

What do we mean by the best available external clinical evidence? We mean the findings of patient-centred clinical research into the accuracy and precision of assessment and intervention. In mental health, a 'test' (as compared with a lab test in physical health) is a summation of the elements obtained from the clinical assessment. These include family history, current mental state and the type and characteristics of risks and benefits that a young person is currently exposed to. The clinical assessment also tests the value of any within-person prognostic markers that can inform the likelihood of therapeutic success, such as the severity of the presenting mental illness and whether there is a history of suicidality and self-harm.

Reviewing and incorporating changes in the ongoing external clinical evidence is important because it can invalidate previously accepted components of assessment that have contributed to the existing treatment plan. Taking into account the therapeutic impact of new changes in the external influences on mental state, such as family breakdown or reconstitution, should replace prior knowledge. This is because new information constitutes likely key prognostic markers for treatment response that are probably more powerful than prior knowledge about the same factors. More powerful prognostic markers mean greater precision in management and care for the individual patient, together with improved effectiveness of treatment. This is of course a critical central outcome of good delivery of evidence-informed and evidence-based care.

A Council for Training in Evidence-Based Behavioral Practice (EBBP) was constituted in the USA, which included experts in medicine, nursing, psychology, social work, public health and information science. The Council introduced a transdisciplinary model of EBBP (see Figure 2.1 based on this model) which delineated the necessary competencies. This was supported by launching www.ebbp.org, a free online training site for understanding the evidence base in the behavioural sciences.

The four-circle model we use to denote EBBP captures the inputs to EBBP from a broad set of evidence-sensitive domains, which include the following:

(i)   From scientific medicine and psychology comes the emphasis on best available research evidence.

(ii) From nursing and mental health practitioners comes acknowledgement that health decision-making needs to be consensual, with patient experience taken into account wherever possible and shared collaboratively. This will best reflect the characteristics, preferences, experiences and values of individual, family and community stakeholders.

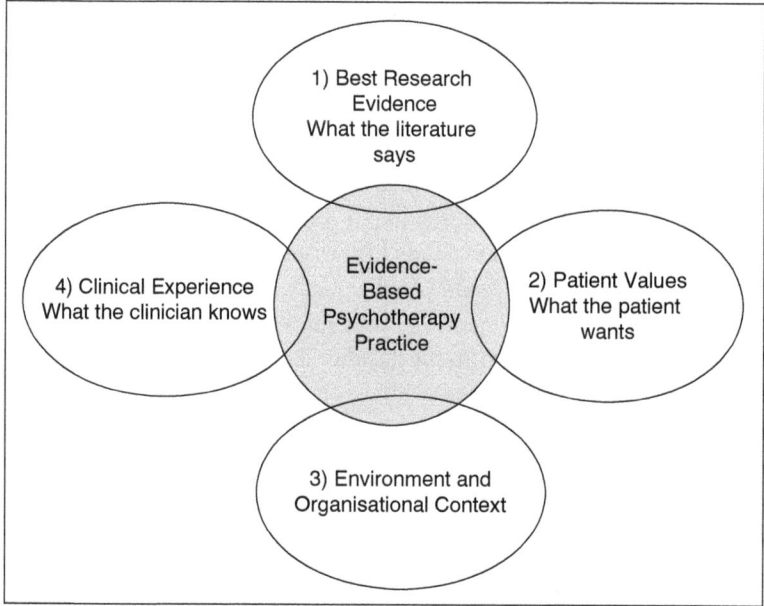

Figure 2.1 The four principles of evidence-based psychotherapy practice

(iii) From public health comes recognition that resource considerations necessarily figure prominently in health decisions, and thus warrant their own circle reflecting financial, logistical, linguistic and other issues constraining access to care.

(iv) From social work comes the insight that decision-making, both clinical and policy-related, about health unfolds in an institutional, organisational and cultural context that inevitably shapes which strategies are likely to be acceptable and effective.

A set of learning points was espoused for the EBBP practice process as follows:

(i)   searching for evidence
(ii) systematic reviews of the evidence
(iii) RCTs
(iv) critical appraisal of the evidence
(v)   shared decision-making with individuals/clients
(vi) collaborative decision-making with communities and key stakeholder perspectives
(vii) implementation science to embed practice change

An Evidence Base for Psychotherapy with Mentally Ill Adolescents

We believe that psychotherapy with mentally ill adolescents should be selected on the available evidence base. When considering what we know regarding psychotherapies for adolescents, it is clear that we have to take a number of differing strands of evidence into account, as currently there are few clear-cut findings that point to a definitive method or set of techniques to be used. Currently, we do not have enough of an evidence base to definitively answer the question of what treatment works best for which adolescent patient. The psychotherapist working with adolescents therefore has to give weight to the lines of evidence that are currently available and come to a clinical decision about treatment knowing that they are likely to define a 'best estimate' for the way forward in many cases. The evidence base to be considered should include findings from RCTs that support a treatment modality for the diagnosis or difficulties presenting in the patient; systematic reviews and metanalyses of trials are important as they can assess where a treatment has been reproduced across such studies, improving the confidence that this may be helpful or indeed the treatment of choice.

As noted in Figure 2.1, evidence should also be drawn from other available written communications; these can include well-written case reports, qualitative experiences of therapists, patient experiences of therapy and collections of cases considered similar enough to be studied as a group. Qualitative research provides much-needed information at the level of the individual: this can include the direct experiences of young people in therapy, those of the parent/s and other family members and also those of the therapists themselves.

Psychotherapists should, however, also use evidence from clinical experience obtained by reflecting on their individual clinical expertise and that of their colleagues. One of the many values of supervision is the ability to draw on the experience as well as the expertise of others, especially those with more years in treating adolescent mental illness. Finally, crucially, the evidence should include listening to and collaborating with their patients in order to arrive at the best clinical assessment that can lead to a collaboratively agreed treatment plan. Without considering clinical experience, practice risks becoming subordinate to evidence that may actually be inapplicable, inappropriate or unacceptable tov the individual patient. Without current best research evidence, however, practice risks becoming rapidly out of date, determined by and overly reliant on the therapist's beliefs, possibly to the detriment of patients.

The multiple sources of evidence and how best to collate and use them may create uncertainty for psychotherapists who are looking to improve clinical decision-making and practical therapeutic skills. Indeed, we conjecture that many busy mental health specialists are likely to avoid evidence that may disrupt their existing therapeutic beliefs, especially if they have experience-based individual patient outcomes that were successful. The centrality of applying the evidence base to a particular case is, however, a practice essential. This is best obtained by peer supervision and support amongst practitioners in a clinical service that has a programme of maintaining an evidence-based practice.

Clinical Value of Evidence-Based Approach to Therapy

For the practising therapist, Figure 2.2 outlines a five-steps approach to collating the evidence base to ensure good clinical decision-making.

The therapist in their first meeting with the adolescent and family is setting out to form the best collaborative working relationship with the young person. We discuss the characteristics of relationship-building and its purpose in subsequent chapters. In brief therapy, a collaborative working relationship is the best relational stance to have with a young person and achieving this will likely occupy the content of this first session and be affirmed in successive

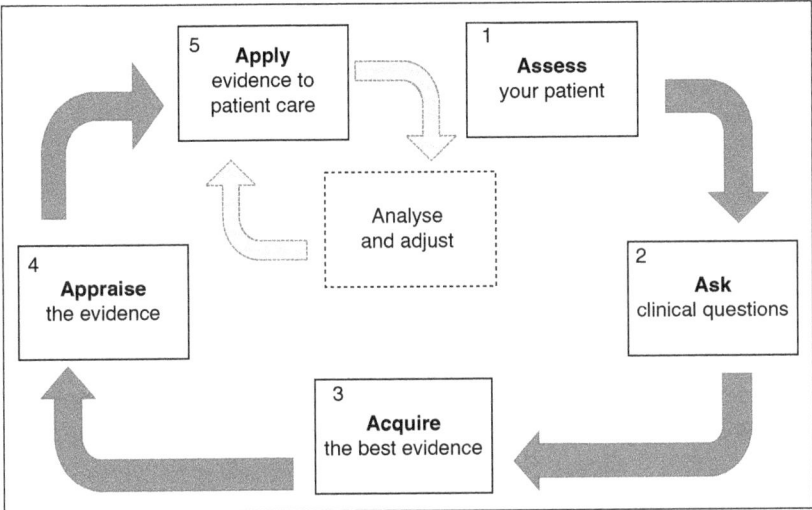

Figure 2.2 Steps of an evidence-based process

meetings. The early purpose of this collaboration is for the therapist to ask clinical questions about the current mental state and frame these in the social and personal context of the adolescent together with a compilation of risks and protective factors, noting those that may moderate treatment response. The third step in the evidence-based process map described in Figure 2.2 is acquiring the best evidence to inform the subsequent formulation of a treatment plan. This is likely to involve discussions with supervisors and peers and attention to the literature on clinical effects. The fourth step is to critically appraise all the evidence (research, clinical information, context and the adolescent's perceptions and experience, available resources). Fifth, apply the evidence by emphasising and engaging in collaborative health decision-making with the adolescent and, where appropriate, with parents or guardians and, if required, other stakeholders.

These five steps are practised through an *active information exchange* with the adolescent. This means conversation, clarification and discussion of life experiences, current social and family contexts, an agreed understanding of current problems and an estimate of the strengths of the young person and their environment. The assessment will include evaluating the role of health care disparities and specific stressors (e.g. housing, education status, major life events). One key goal of evidence-based psychotherapy is to maximise patient choice about options and prioritise this wherever possible, including the decision not to proceed.

We note that evidence-based psychotherapy is more ethical to practise, potentially maximising the opportunities for positive effects and minimising the probability of the negative effects discussed below. By incorporating both quantitative and qualitative research into clinical practice, providers use research-driven evidence rather than relying solely on personal opinion. Using empirical evidence reduces opinion-based bias such as recalling only successes.

Negative Effects of Psychotherapies

There is general agreement that psychotherapies can also be associated with a worsening of presenting symptoms and behavioural functions in 5% to 20% of cases across the life-course. A number of reviews and opinion articles over the past 20 years have agreed that students learning to become psychotherapists should be trained in the recognition, evaluation and documentation of side effects. Therapists should learn how to take possible negative consequences into account when planning treatment. Currently, however, there is neither an agreed definition of negative effects nor a set of standard practice principles that therapists should adhere to in order to reduce the risk of such effects. Here we describe and collate the current thoughts of experts and patients regarding the potentially harmful or negative effects of psychotherapy. Almost all this information has been obtained from studies and surveys of psychotherapy for adult patients [4].

Clinical Deterioration

Therapists can observe and assess clinical deterioration characterised by a worsening of the presenting signs and symptoms and/or a decline in behavioural and social functions since the initial assessment. Clinical deterioration can be defined as a negative change between two time points in presenting signs and symptoms and/or associated behavioural functions. Such a change can be clinically estimated through a session-by-session evaluation, with the therapist taking time to estimate progress from the patient perspective.

In practice, this is likely to involve a period of time at the beginning of the session during which the young person is asked about how they have been since their last visit. A systematic re-evaluation of their mental state and psychosocial functions will allow an estimation of change to be revealed through collaboration with the young person. For adolescents in therapy, other informants such as parents, siblings and school staff can also be asked for their perception of progress and change, with the permission of the young person.

The term 'negative effects' is, however, more global than examining for between-session clinical deterioration. Negative effects also include potentially harmful, adverse or unwanted consequences of psychotherapy. Both adverse and unwanted events are situations where the patient experiences an unforeseen and undesirable effect that is directly due to the treatment.

Unwanted Events

The wider assessment of negative side effects can start with the recording of unwanted events. These are events that occur parallel to or in the context of treatment and are burdensome to the patient or others in the immediate environment. Unwanted effects are not dependent on clinical deterioration in the current mental state. In psychotherapy, for example, crying may be unavoidable or even necessary and create a temporary worsening of the mind in order to regain a better mental state subsequently. This notion of recovery involving a transient increase in burden is not confined to psychotherapy: think of the rehabilitation of movement in a limb that requires considerable effort in learning to walk again after a fracture. Mental recovery likewise can be effortful, requiring strategies that may be unwanted but are of value because they enhance a return to well-being.

From an evidence-based perspective, therapists must maintain an awareness of and inform themselves about new treatments that may reduce unwanted effects. For example, a new treatment for depression that has the same clinical effect but carries fewer negative effects should be considered potentially more valuable than current practice and perhaps more ethically appropriate.

Adverse Treatment Reactions

Adverse treatment reactions are negative undesirable events which are likely or known to be caused by the treatment. There are three types of adverse effects to be considered when planning a psychotherapy with young people.

Side Effects

Side effects are unexpected adverse reactions, which are likely directly caused by a correct treatment. Side effects that occur routinely when applying a special type of treatment constitute the 'side effect profile' of that treatment. These regularly occurring side effects must be taken into account in planning the therapy and patients should be informed about the side effect profile before starting treatment. Currently, we have no clear-cut understanding of what side effects profile may accrue from psychotherapy with adolescents. Therapists are advised to pay particular attention to an unexpected deterioration in mental state and psychosocial functions or a loss of improvement, as these may be indicative of side effects even when the treatment is considered as the best to be given for this patient. In contrast to adverse effects from a correct treatment, application of an incorrect treatment is likely to evoke both side effects and clinical deterioration. Therapists are advised to always reflect on their treatment choice before implementation and wherever possible be a member of a professional peer group where treatment choice and progress can be discussed.

Contraindications

Contraindications are serious side effects that must be expected in special types of patients if the treatment is applied. Here the treatment cannot be applied because there is a pre-existing component or condition in the young person and/or their family that prevents the efficacious implementation of the psychotherapy. Again, we remain very unclear as to which contraindications are likely to emerge from different types of psychotherapies applied to adolescents with mental illness.

Therapist Effects

Finally, unlike pharmacological treatments, prescribing psychotherapy means that the therapist is an explicitly active agent in treatment. How one functions as a therapist therefore influences treatment efficacy and effectiveness. This unique position means that the therapist's actions are part of the prescription of the treatment and therefore may exert negative as well as positive effects on treatment response. The likeliest area where negative effects of the therapist's behaviour may arise is in the relationship with the young person and/or their family/carers. The commonly reported areas of concern are 'non-compliance' of the patient with treatment; strains in the patient–therapist relationship; patient–therapist relationship distortions, including therapy dependency. We do not know enough about how or how much these therapist–patient relation factors exert a negative effect on treatment outcomes with young people, but they appear very important from observations of routine practice. We consider that, with the current lack of direct evidence, abnormalities in therapist–patient relationships could be considered a component of the adverse side effects profile of psychotherapies.

REFERENCES

1. Cochrane AL. *Effectiveness and Efficiency: Random Reflections on Health Services.* London: The Nuffield Trust, 1972.
2. Spring B, Hoffman S, Steglitz J. History and process of evidence-based practice in mental health. In Dimidjian IS, editor. *Evidence-Based Practice in Action.* New York: Guilford Press, 2019. pp. 9–27.

3. Sackett DL, Rosenberg WM, Gray JA, Haynes RB, Richardson WS. Evidence based medicine: what it is and what it isn't. *BMJ.* 1996;312(7023):71–2.

4. Cook SC, Schwartz AC, Kaslow NJ. Evidence-based psychotherapy: advantages and challenges. *Neurotherapeutics.* 2017;14(3):537–45.

3 Evolving the BPI Method

In Chapter 1 we described the emergence of the concept of adolescence in the early twentieth century and how it represented a new and developmentally sensitive period of ongoing mental maturation. We also noted that the talking cures were fast gaining a foothold in developed societies and adolescents were beginning to be a focus of these interventions, this being due to the clear-cut increases in mental health difficulties and emergent mental illnesses in the second decade of life. The theories and techniques of the psychotherapies were, until the 1970s, relatively uninfluenced by the emergence of the concept of adolescence and its implications for mind-brain maturation. This implies that very little of what we know about adolescents and their mental states has been taken into account when devising a talking treatment for young people. The reality has been that psychotherapy methods developed top-down (adult to adolescent) or occasionally bottom-up (child to adolescent) and have been practised with a modest evidence base at best, as described in Chapter 2. With increasing knowledge about human development and psychopathology in the second decade of life, new theory and perhaps new practices are required to improve the effectiveness of mental health interventions in the adolescent years.

Brief Psychosocial Intervention

The Value of Good Clinical Care As a Key Component of Intervention

Anxiety and depression are common mental problems in the adolescent age range, with a higher incidence than at any other period in the life-course. Furthermore, talking therapies have expanded enormously in the management of mental illness in young people. Despite the availability of literally hundreds of therapies over the past 30 years, there has been virtually no change for the better in the outcome of depressed adolescents and new interventions are likely required [1]. One of the key observations is that, when any of the well-tried psychotherapies are compared with good clinical care, the differences in outcomes are much smaller than when the new intervention is compared with no treatment at all. Doing something active is clearly better for the patient than doing nothing, but what the ingredients are that reduce mental difficulties and improve well-being and behavioural function is not known. Indeed, the mechanisms of action of CBT, probably the most frequently used group of interventions for mental health problems across the life-course, remain unknown.

From the scientific perspective, as RCTs of adolescents referred to mental health clinics have begun to compare active psychotherapies with each other when treating adolescents, we see that the specialised therapy being investigated is often little or no better than structured, manualised, active good clinical care. In general terms, this means that many episodes of mental distress, problems and even full-blown and severe depression and anxiety may be effectively treated with the therapist adhering to common principles that include forming a caring relationship, listening in a non-judgemental manner and offering advice and support about recovery and the future. To date, the results of pragmatic RCTs for depressed adolescents have established that good clinical care delivered by a mental health practitioner working in a specialist clinic for child and adolescent mental health services (CAMHS) is as clinically effective as CBT and short term psychoanalytic psychotherapy [2, 3].

BPI Practice Principles

Brief psychosocial intervention is a treatment based on good structured clinical care, built upon the following principles: (i) collaborative care, (ii) comprehensive assessment/understanding of the person and their mental state, (iii) listening, information-giving, (iv) advising, (v) problem-solving, (vi) safety, (vii) caring and explaining about adolescent depression. These components provide the foundation for the tools required for a comprehensive assessment and engagement of the young person and their parents or carers, as shown in Figure 3.1.

Emphasis is placed on the importance of psychoeducation about depression and action-oriented, goal-focused, interpersonal activities as therapeutic strategies, with a particular emphasis on prosocial behaviours with friends and family. This springs from an expertise-informed understanding of the person and their state of mind, knitting together how the disorder impacts this particular person and their physical relationships and social worlds. Where needed, specific advice can be given on improving and maintaining mental and physical hygiene, engaging in pleasurable activities, maintaining and/or rejoining peer relations, ensuring efficient and effective schoolwork and diminishing solitariness.

As BPI does not require the application of cognitive or reflective analytic techniques, there is no need for discussions of unconscious conflict or any deliberate effort to modify maladaptive models of attachment relationships. Neither is there any detailed focus on directly changing cognitions. Negative

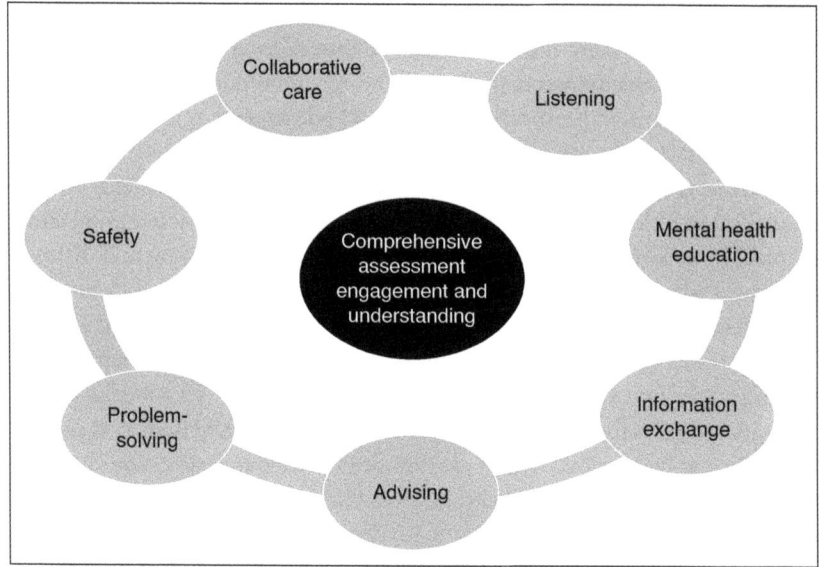

Figure 3.1 BPI practice principles

cognition-driven behaviours are not deconstructed systematically or in detail, as can occur in CBT.

Here we provide brief descriptions of the key BPI practice principles and the associated clinical tools we recommend to achieve the goal of a comprehensive assessment (Figure 3.2). Note that a comprehensive assessment includes therapeutic engagement with and an understanding of the young person from their perspective.

Brief psychosocial intervention is most likely to be clinically effective when a comprehensive assessment is made based on the practice principles shown in Figures 3.1 and 3.2. The suite of clinical tools in Figure 3.2 should be used to achieve the formulation that underpins treatment decision-making. There is no prescribed order for using the clinical tools. Given the probable individual differences between patterns of risk factors associated with clinical presentations, the therapist will need to determine the likeliest best tools to achieve the required assessment and, subsequently, treatment.

Achieving a Comprehensive Assessment

The key element of BPI is a comprehensive, person-centred, holistic assessment of both depth and breadth. From the individual will come the presenting complaints and problems; the therapist must assess the current mental state, any recent life events and difficulties, identify risk and protective factors, obtain

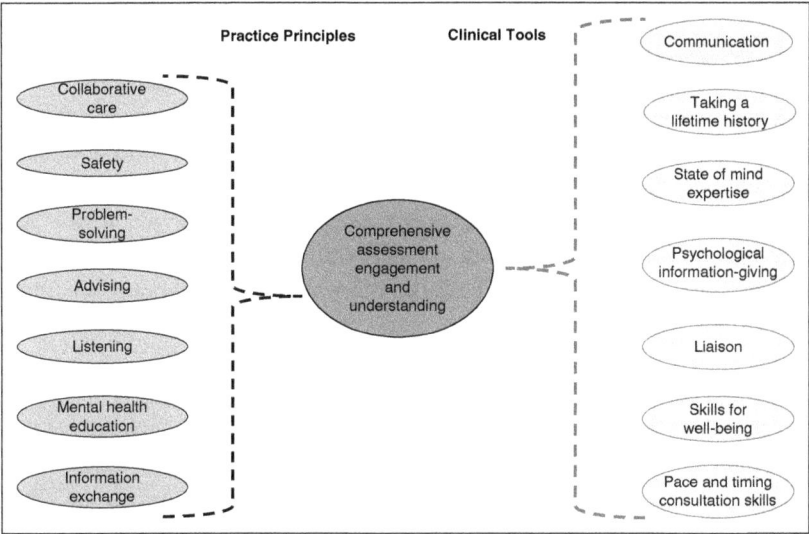

Figure 3.2 Practice principles and their associated clinical tools

the adolescent's perception of their life including friends, family, school/college and local environment and community. A diagnosis based on the presenting signs and symptoms is desirable but not sufficient for a BPI formulation. So too is an evaluation of any co-occurring disorders (comorbidities) and hazardous behaviours, such as self-harming and/or drug and alcohol misuse, and a developmental history. These will help pick up any other risk or indeed protective factors, including any safeguarding issues. Corroborative and additional information from parents and, where appropriate and with consents, from the young person's educational setting is very helpful, where it is available.

Brief psychosocial intervention therapists are likely to select several clinical tools from the available 'toolbox'. Clear communication with the young person is always a prerequisite and promotes a working relationship through which information-giving can occur. Formulations are likely to involve revealing, characterising and explaining mental states to the adolescent, which requires the therapist to utilise state of mind expertise.

Collaborative Care

Collaborative care emerges from making clinical use of good communication, thereby eliciting information. This organises treatment and care, contributing to improved outcomes, and is the core principle on which BPI is based. As well as the aforementioned clinical tools, it may be necessary to use liaison skills with others in the social environment who have an influence on the adolescent's well-being.

In BPI, collaborative care involves the therapist also acting as the adolescent's 'case manager', which is a process that facilitates recommended treatment plans to assure the appropriate care is provided to mentally unwell adolescents.

This dual role ensures that the physical and social context of the young person is incorporated into the delivery of BPI. The probability of a good treatment outcome is enhanced by assessing and evaluating the young person's current physical and social environment: friends, family, school, college, workplace. The 'therapist as case manager' implies that where it is considered involving others may improve outcomes, this can be done. This would be a collaborative decision between the adolescent, their parents/carers and the therapist as case manager.

Listening and Information-Receiving

Eliciting a clinical history about the presenting complaint, the concerns of the young person and their family, their social background and context is a component skill required to obtain information for a complete formulation. This is part of the general therapeutic process of information exchange where the therapist is likely to use many of the clinical tools but will especially find themselves regulating the pace and the timing of the questions they may want to ask to help build a formulation. We recommend the pacing of questions and seeking clarification as a tool for enhancing engagement and understanding (key to a valid formulation). The judicious use of listening and information-gathering using the clinical tools is of considerable value in ensuring collaboration, sharing knowledge and having a dialogue about conjectures and inferences regarding the current mental health of the young person. Brief psychosocial intervention therapists will not 'lose effect' by being patient and considerate in their approach. Indeed, as we have emphasised, helping the adolescent to understand more about their mental state and their immediate social environment substantially contributes to the clinical formulation and is of itself likely to be clinically effective.

Information-Giving, Advising and Problem-Solving

As part of the general process of information exchange noted above, the therapist will provide educative information about mental states and illnesses such as depression. The compassionate and caring approach is retained throughout therapy. This is a framework for providing professional advice, contributing to solving problems in the real world and in the mind of the young person. All the clinical tools can be of assistance but being focused and clear on psychological information-giving, using state of mind expertise and emphasising the value of knowledge and intervention to well-being can, in our view, be particularly valuable here.

Safety and Safeguarding

The young person's safety is paramount at all times. The therapist has, of course, a prime professional duty to do all they can to ensure that the safety of the adolescent is always maintained throughout BPI. Therapist liaison skills will be important in any concerning environmental circumstances.

Formulating the Case

The purpose of the comprehensive assessment described in the previous section is to create a formulation of the case. Clinical formulation was introduced to mental health practice in its present form relatively recently, in the 1970s. It was, however, based on the biopsychosocial framework proposed by Adolf Meyer in the 1920s. Meyer's conceptualisations were themselves a modern version of a twelfth-century thesis proposing moderation and a healthy lifestyle for a balanced life, principles emphasised and reaffirmed in modern psychological medicine practice [4]. A clinical formulation is, in essence, a concise summary of the origins, nature and context of a person's problems and strengths, together with an opinion on what may go wrong in the future and what steps should be taken to improve matters. We consider BPI to be a person-centred, holistic and recovery-oriented intervention approach that is a logical and pragmatic clinical consequence of taking this biopsychosocial approach to mood-related mental health difficulties presenting in adolescents.

A formulation is more than just restating the facts. It is an exercise in clinical reasoning, one that requires making judgements and, from there, decisions. The decisions include the choice of techniques and tools required for the intervention. The philosophical stance includes that of the clinician as scientist testing 'hypotheses' derived from the formulation. Thereafter, reviewing 'progress' and amending the 'treatment path' informed by regular patient and parent/carer feedback, including ROMs (routine outcome measures). This key element (formulation) of the first part of engagement in BPI has six underpinning principles that are adapted from general mental health practice (Figure 3.3) [5]:

(i)   *Chronological*: the story should be mostly in the sequence in which it occurred.
(ii) *Concise*: the prose should be clear and accessible, without jargon.
(iii) *Complete*: should insufficient information or understanding accrue and prevent good enough understanding of presenting concerns, then this should be stated. An account of what still needs to be elicited and why this may be of potential value should be given.
(iv) *Practical*: common sense should never be lost in a description of a young person's mental health difficulties and social history.

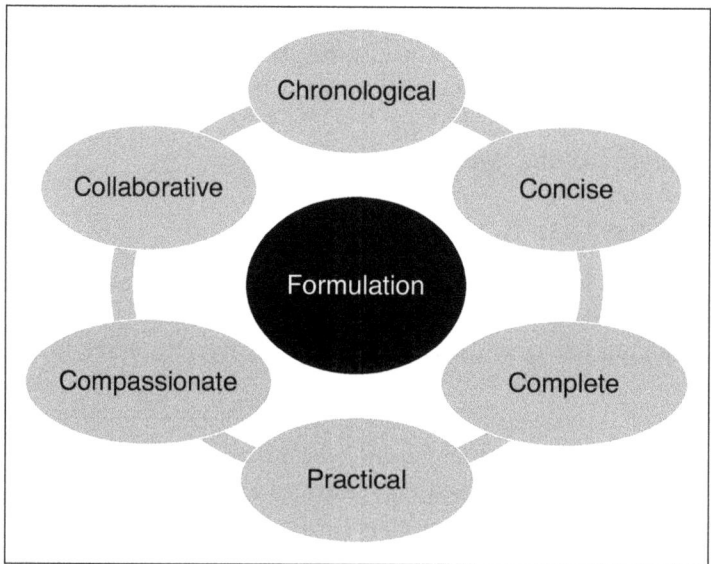

Figure 3.3 Guiding principles for clinical formulation of a case

(v) *Compassionate*: compassion, a person-centred approach, should be palpable throughout the process. The working explanation for the presenting problem and related difficulties should assume that they are the products of the young person's life experiences and difficulties.

(vi) *Collaborative*: the young person and, where possible, family and carers and, where appropriate along with consents, school/college could or even should all be involved.

From the clinical formulation derived from the comprehensive clinical assessment will come a plan for case management and clinical treatment. Further details and applications of therapy are discussed in subsequent chapters.

Outline of BPI Intervention

Brief psychosocial intervention has a tripartite strategy of:

(i) *Pedagogy*: the provision of information and understanding about mental states and how mental illnesses emerge and their effects on behaviour.

(ii) *Social Prescribing*: the use of prosocial and personal activities to reduce misperceptions of the social environment, foster a reduction in mental illness and promote well-being.

iii) *Habilitation*: supporting and encouraging learning about mental states, prosocial gains and general physical and emotional well-being and reinforcing gains and personal competences – a recovery orientation.

The delivery of BPI places emphasis on the importance of psychoeducation about mental states and depression in particular. It is action-oriented and goal-focused, incorporating interpersonal activities as therapeutic strategies.

To summarise, specific advice is given on understanding normal and abnormal mental states, improving and maintaining mental and physical hygiene, engaging in pleasurable social and personal activities, engaging with and maintaining schoolwork and peer relations and the importance of diminishing solitariness.

Delivering BPI

A BPI operating plan consists of up to 12 sessions of around 45 minutes each, delivered on average over 20 to 24 weeks. In reality, adolescents on average complete about 50% of the sessions as shown in Figure 4.3. This is consistent with all psychotherapies given for adolescents. For BPI, inclusion of family/parents/guardians in sessions is to be expected when deemed clinically of value to improving the mental health of the adolescent patient. There are likely to be up to four such sessions with the adolescent in the room. Some parents/guardians will benefit from updates after each session or want to gain further clarity for themselves about mental illness and the aims of BPI for their children. These are important psychoeducative elements for parents/guardians and BPI sees them as such, to be carried out wherever possible with the collaborative agreement of the young patient. Liaison with external agencies and personnel (e.g. teachers, social care workers and peer groups) is commonly undertaken as part of the case management element integral to BPI.

As noted above, case management is a key component of BPI therapeutics and not merely a passive support process used during one-to-one clinical conversations. This emphasises that BPI has an overarching social-relational framework even when the focus of the intervention is on the adolescent alone. There are three key elements to 'case management' as part of therapy:

Interpersonal Effectiveness

This psychosocial element refers to the ability to interact with others. Adolescents' interpersonal skills are evolving as they extend their social and personal networks beyond their immediate family. In case management, the therapist's interpersonal effectiveness is needed to engage the mentally ill adolescent in conversation about themselves, their lives and experiences, their perceptions of their mental state and, of course, their interpersonal personal effectiveness. The therapist has the objective of engaging, relaxing, building trust and developing a working alliance through their interpersonal effectiveness skills.

Understanding of Mental States

Utilising these interpersonal skills will permit the therapist to characterise and evaluate the current mental state: the moods, thoughts, feelings and sensations that the adolescent has in the present and in the recent past (the last two weeks especially). A formal assessment of the mental state will elicit sufficient information to judge the extent to which social functions and performance with friends and family and in school/college settings are likely to be associated with the current state of mind of the young person. We consider that an efficient mental state is one where incoming information from the environment is appraised and assigned a value that activates a mental state and subsequently this [value + mental state] is cleared to memory. Mental states that do not clear to memory are occupying mental space and preventing efficient mental processing.

Social Activation and Problem-Solving

Finally, case management will depend on the therapist judging the extent to which psychoeducative explanations, prosocial prescribing and goal-focused and problem-oriented solutions should be used as interventions for current difficulties. Judging the current competence of the young person will assist in determining problem analyses, which include identifying, prioritising and selecting alternatives and implementing a solution through collaborative methods. The three domains of BPI practice are summarised in Figure 3.4.

BPI Summary

Brief psychosocial intervention is a formalised and manualised psychotherapy that emerged from long-standing clinical practice in child and adolescent mental health services in the UK. It is therefore a set of strategies that developed from observing and evaluating the pragmatic effects of the interventions that have been tried, used for many years and now tested through RCTs. The current method is a brief intervention, likely to be between 4 and 11 sessions, that is active and looking for effects in three domains: (i) returning the atypical mental state to its prior more adaptive, efficient and effective state, (ii) using the social

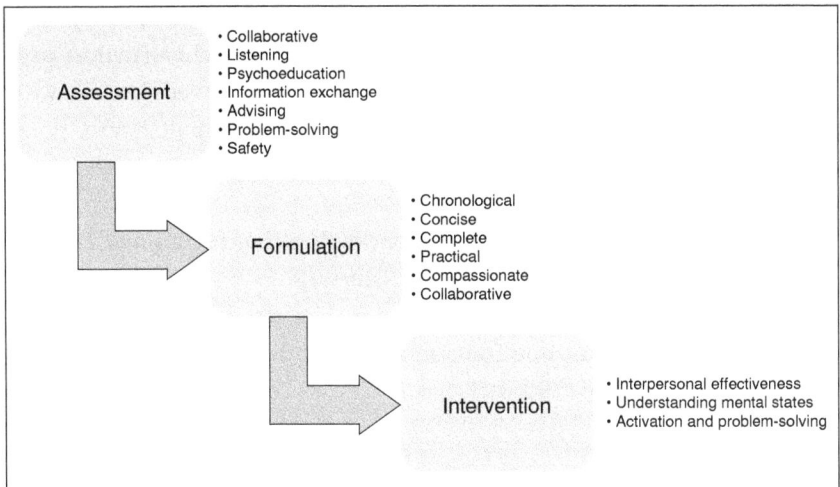

Figure 3.4 BPI domains of practice

and the personal environment to effect better behavioural functioning in the world, which can involve friends, family, school, learning performance, hobbies and achievements, (iii) learning and embedding skills to reduce subsequent risks and/or reduce the liability of further episodes of mental health difficulties.

Brief psychosocial intervention is a clinically effective intervention for depressed adolescents with comorbid anxieties and self-harming behaviours. Remember, however, that it is no more effective than any other psychotherapy for adolescents with these difficulties. It is therefore a further clinically useful intervention that could be made available to adolescent mental health services to expand capacity or consolidate the therapeutic skills of those practising in child and adolescent mental health clinics.

REFERENCES

1. Eckshtain D, Kuppens S, Ugueto A, Ng MY, Vaughn-Coaxum R, Corteselli K et al. Meta-analysis: 13-year follow-up of psychotherapy effects on youth depression. *J Am Acad Child Adolesc Psychiatry*. 2020;59(1):45–63.

2. Goodyer I, Dubicka B, Wilkinson P, Kelvin R, Roberts C, Byford S et al. Selective serotonin reuptake inhibitors (SSRIs) and routine specialist care with and without cognitive behaviour therapy in adolescents with major depression: randomised controlled trial. *BMJ*. 2007;335(7611):142.

3. Goodyer IM, Reynolds S, Barrett B, Byford S, Dubicka B, Hill J et al. Cognitive behavioural therapy and short-term psychoanalytical psychotherapy versus a brief psychosocial intervention in adolescents with unipolar major depressive disorder (IMPACT): a multicentre, pragmatic, observer-blind, randomised controlled superiority trial. *Lancet Psychiatry*. 2017;4(2):109–19.
4. Bolton D, Gillett G. *The Biopsychosocial Model of Health and Disease*. Cham, Switzerland: Palgrave Macmillan, 2019.
5. Baird J, Hyslop A, Macfie M, Stocks R, Van der Kleij T. Clinical formulation: where it came from, what it is and why it matters. *BJPsych Advances*. 2017;23(2):95–103.

4 The Evidence Base for BPI

Brief psychosocial intervention was first used as a non-manualised reference treatment for depressed adolescents receiving the antidepressant fluoxetine with or without CBT. Both the treatment groups received the forerunner of BPI, specialist clinical care, as their general clinical support. The surprise was that CBT provided no added value over fluoxetine and specialist clinical care by the end of the study, which was only a short-term outcome of some 28 weeks [1]. This was the first finding that specialist clinical care provided by psychiatrists and mental health nurses to depressed adolescents may be as clinically effective as specialised psychological treatments such as CBT.

An interesting consequence of this study was to ask: what exactly did the therapists do when delivering specialist clinical care and how was it delivered? The research practitioners who delivered BPI in this trial were not formally trained in any specific therapy nor were they especially experienced in the mental health care of adolescents, although they had a minimum of around 6 to 12 months working in child and adolescent mental health services. We conjectured that it was likely that the general education and orientation of their clinical training and supervision, especially about psychotherapy, would have influenced the method used with the adolescents in the clinic.

The study also had a preliminary phase to the treatment trial proper: individuals whose illness may have already been in a recovery phase and were therefore likely to enter clinical remission regardless of the available treatments were offered up to three sessions of mental health education about depression and the likely natural course and history of mental illnesses emerging during adolescence. Again, to our surprise, several moderately to severely depressed adolescents referred to outpatients for the trial responded to this apparently simple information-giving and explanation of depression without any more intervention, including no fluoxetine. Considering these results and the clinical observations that accompanied them, the implications for treatment were that there may be a valid psychosocial intervention to distil, characterise and implement from 'non-specific' specialist clinical care. We conjectured that such an emerging intervention could be delivered by trained mental health staff.

Even if this were possible, however, it was unclear whether this pragmatic clinical intervention was in fact as good as proven treatments with known efficacy and effectiveness, such as CBT. The opportunity to test the clinical effectiveness of a new treatment based on specialist clinical care presented itself through funding obtained for a second RCT, which investigated whether the specialist therapies of CBT and STPP were superior in treating adolescents with major depression compared with a reference treatment based on specialist clinical care, now refined, manualised and renamed as 'brief psychosocial intervention'. This new study was undertaken across three regions of England: North London, East Anglia and the North-West. Since there was already evidence that CBT is clinically effective in reducing depressive symptoms, the primary objective was to determine whether CBT was superior to STPP in maintaining expected reductions from treatment in depressive symptoms for up to a year following the end of treatment.

Secondly, we wanted to determine whether either of the more specialist treatments was superior to a reference treatment of BPI, which was shorter, delivered by routine mental health psychiatry and nursing and at this point had no systematic evidence to support its effectiveness in maintaining reductions in symptoms in the year following treatment.

The study used 15 routine NHS child and adolescent mental health services receiving referrals from primary care, schools and social services, to provide participants for this study. Each region (North London, East Anglia and North-West England) provided five such services and 465 depressed adolescent patients between the ages of 11 and 17 years were recruited from them. All gave written informed consent, as did their parents/carers. Patients were randomised to one of the three treatments. The outline of the trial design is shown in Figure 4.1.

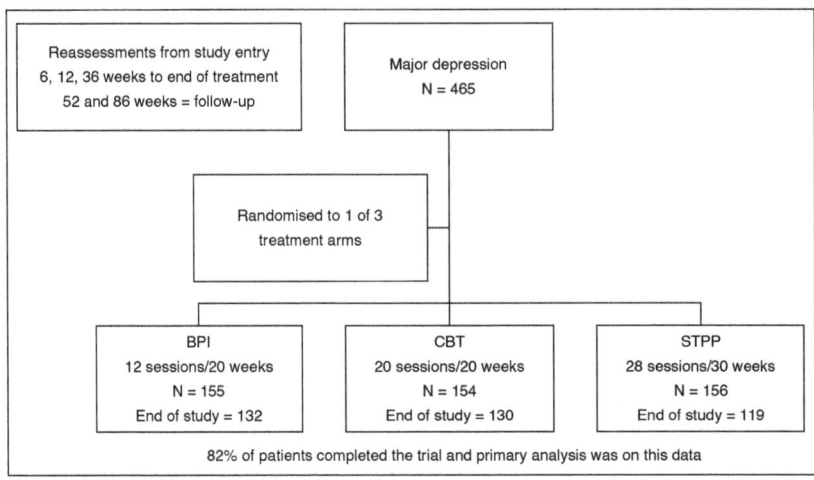

Figure 4.1 Improving mood with psychoanalytic and cognitive behaviour therapy

The treatments were delivered by the following practitioners:

BPI: child and adolescent consultant and trainee psychiatrists and mental health nurses.

CBT: clinical psychologists or other professionals with post-qualification training in CBT.

STPP: child and adolescent psychotherapists and trainees in their last year.

All therapists were supervised by senior staff within the three treatment domains.

The primary outcome measure was self-reported depression sum scores at each of the nominal reassessment time points. Level of psychosocial impairment and anxiety symptoms were secondary outcome measures. The trial result for the primary outcome (depression symptom sum scores) is shown in Figure 4.2.

The figure shows that the self-reported depression symptom mean sum scores (the error bars index the standard deviations) by treatment group over time were no different from each other's scores at any time point over the course of the study. This can be observed during treatment (0 to 40 weeks) and over the follow-up post-treatment period (41 to 100 weeks). The conclusion drawn from this main result was that all three therapies are equally effective in maintaining symptom reductions and improving psychosocial functions up to a year after treatment. Brief psychosocial intervention was shown to be equally effective

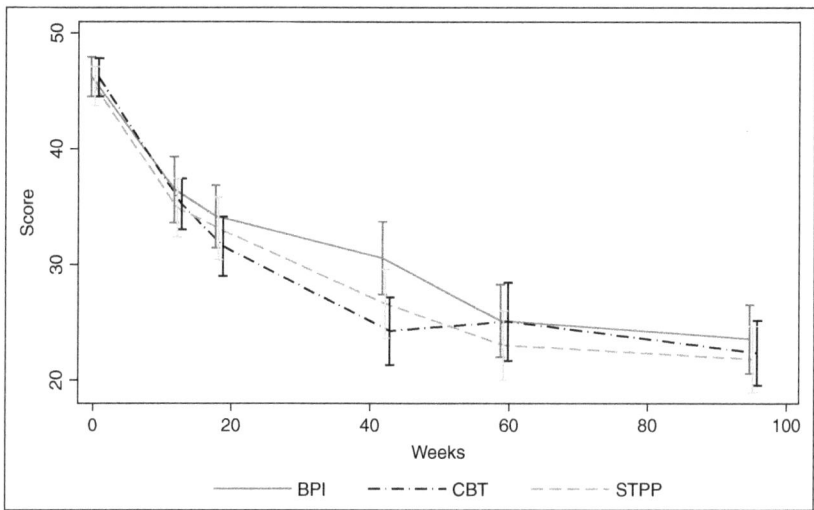

Figure 4.2 Self-reported depression sum scores over the study

during both the treatment phase and the follow-up phase. Neither CBT nor STPP was superior to each other or to BPI in terms of effecting a treatment response or maintaining improvements after treatment had finished. These findings confirmed that BPI is clinically effective and, together with STPP, provides alternative therapies to CBT for adolescents presenting with depression.

Importantly the effects of all three of the psychological therapies extend to comorbid diagnoses and non-depressive symptoms at presentation. Psychological treatments for depression, including BPI, are therefore transdiagnostic, being able to reduce anxiety symptoms, personal impairments and self-harm and antisocial difficulties at presentation [2, 3].

Furthermore, at a follow-up one year post treatment around 16% of the patients had relapsed, with their self-reported depression scores at or near original baseline entry levels [4]. Interestingly, all patients responded initially so treatment non-response does not appear to emerge until 12 to 18 weeks and after some 3 to 5 sessions of treatment with any therapy. It is important to remember that, taking all studies of psychological treatment of depression into account, the likelihood is around 1 in 5 adolescents who enter therapy will show signs of relapse by 12 to 18 weeks, which could be after 4 to 6 sessions of treatment. A further striking feature was the completion of only around 50% of the therapy sessions initially planned by the relevant manual guidelines, noted in Figure 4.3, which gave an 84% remission rate, defined as having less than 50% of depression symptom sum scores by the end of the study. These were recorded in 391 of the 465 depressed patients. Overall, 80.7% of patients received 11 sessions or fewer.

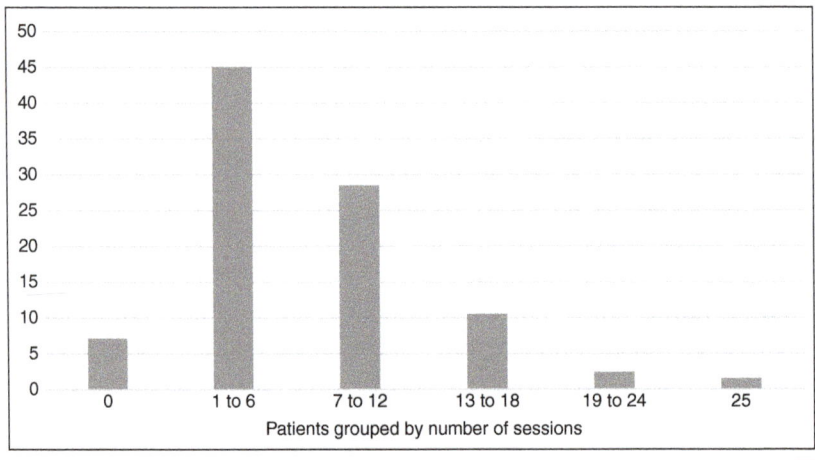

Figure 4.3 Number of BPI sessions delivered to depressed adolescents

The median number of BPI sessions given to depressed adolescents was 6 with an interquartile range of 4 to 11. The figure shows that seven patients declined any treatment after entering the study. The majority (45.1%) received 1 to 6 sessions. The number of sessions did not correlate with depressive symptoms or personal impairment at the end of treatment or at the final follow-up one year later. This suggests that treatments were titrated by the therapists in collaboration with the client's experiences of therapy and progress, consistent with the notion of personalised treatment. Further, in adolescents early end of treatment may be an indicator of good progress. Having said this, it must be recognised that very early non-attendance – that is, missing a session in the first three – is associated with subsequent desistance-withdrawal without progress and therefore can be considered a clinical warning sign for potential non-response [5].

Dose Response

A key feature of modern therapeutics is that interventions are designed to reduce mental symptoms and psychosocial impairments as outcomes. There are, however, no agreed clinical standards regarding how psychotherapies should be practised. Perhaps a key set of standards for psychotherapy with adolescents should be:

(i)   specifying the dose (currently defined as the number and duration of sessions) required to effect clinical remission for different mental illnesses
(ii) describing the expected negative effects of treatment
(iii) defining the prescribing principles, including dose per unit time, total dose duration and withdrawal of therapy guidelines.

Studying dose response and developing dose-response models are central to determining 'safe', 'hazardous' and 'beneficial' levels and dosages for psychotherapies. This has yet to be done for any psychotherapies practised on adolescents with depression or indeed any other mental illness.

The Patient's Experience of BPI

Interviewing depressed adolescents who received BPI about the experience of therapy gives an insight into how the adolescent perceived the intervention and what in their view was key in their mental and behavioural improvement. This information was achieved through a qualitative study using face-to-face interviewing of five adolescents. They were purposively selected as good-outcome cases following BPI and the interviews focused on understanding their experiences of overcoming depression. This qualitative study analysed the written transcripts using five audiotaped interviews. Four central themes emerged as shown in Figure 4.4.

Being Heard and Feeling Safe

This construct was expressed as the therapist making the adolescent feel 'at home' when in therapy. Here the therapist is providing an environment within which the adolescent can adaptively converse. This safe space allows information exchange to occur that is relevant and important to the young person; it creates interpersonal value, leading to trust and improved confidence within the adolescent. These are important components for the effectiveness of BPI and are likely common to all evidence-based therapies used with depressed adolescents [6].

Collaborative Working Is Enhancing Therapy

The second theme of collaborative work in therapy raised by the adolescent feedback is completely consistent with the practice principles delineated and discussed in Chapters 3 and 5. This collaborative notion is likely a common therapeutic principle for conversational therapies with adolescents. Indeed shared decision-making and collaboration are preferred by adolescents as they enable them to embrace an active role in therapy. In good-outcome BPI, adolescents experienced clinicians facilitating the discovery of their experiences through curiosity, active listening, using their expertise sensitively and being attuned to their affective states and pace in sessions. The type of collaboration being sought during BPI is around the adolescent's engagement. It is likely to be

'Being heard and feeling safe'.

'Collaborative working is enhancing therapy'.

'Gaining a different perspective on oneself and relationships'.

'A positive therapeutic relationship'.

Figure 4.4 Core themes associated with being a BPI treatment responder

effortful for them and a prelude to them then engaging in more positive-adaptive prosocial, educational and personal behaviours. This therapist–adolescent partnership facilitates improving the current mental state.

Gaining a Different Perspective on Oneself and Relationships

The third theme describes adolescents gaining a different perspective on their mental state of depression and associated life experiences, through techniques used in BPI. This is a key psychoeducational task: aiding the young people to distinguish between their normal selves and illness-related mental states, as discussed earlier. Therapists help adolescents to distinguish between different forms of mental states by learning to recognise in themselves when the content and function of their mental state are atypical: in such circumstances their current mental state is 'not their friend' and likely to be maladaptive. The adolescents reported giving much value to talking about their lives with their therapist. The *information exchange* process, with clarification and information from the therapist, mattered to them.

Using the BPI practice principles and the clinical tools can facilitate a different perspective on their life experiences and their understanding of their depressed mental state. In this theme emerging from the qualitative study findings, there is a clear suggestion that adolescents bring an expectation to the clinic that therapy will provide a space for talking, helping them get a new perspective (therapist–patient collaborative expertise) on their problems.

A Positive Therapeutic Relationship

The fourth theme emphasises the critical value of the active stance of the BPI therapist for good outcomes. Actively working to develop a positive therapeutic relationship is closely linked to increased client engagement and positive treatment outcomes. This may be because taking a proactive approach enhances the adolescent's experience of being heard and feeling safe, thereby creating the therapeutic conditions for information exchange.

How Might BPI Work to Improve Mental State and Well-Being?

In the field of psychotherapy, the term 'mechanism' refers to an explanation of how conversation-based interventions translate into biological (i.e. psychological and/or physiological) processes that lead to the desired outcome. The mechanism likely consists of activating events, experienced in the mind, that are responsible for the change. Such activations are then the reasons why change occurs and explain how change comes about.

Despite the vast growth in psychotherapies over the past 60 years, with several hundred psychotherapeutic models or techniques described and in use, we remain unclear exactly *why* any one of these works to bring about positive change in the mind and behaviour. Brief psychosocial intervention is no exception and currently we do not understand how improvements in current mental state and associated behaviour are brought about.

The rest of this chapter is given over to our current theorising of how possible BPI-related mechanisms may bring about therapeutic change.

Is There a Common Therapeutic Mechanism for Brief Psychotherapies?

Within RCTs for depressed adolescents, therapies that are theoretically distinct, such as CBT and psychoanalytic psychotherapy, deliver very similar clinical outcomes [7]. The finding that different therapies give similar results suggests there may be some intervention features whose mechanistic effects operate through a single process or set of processes common to all treatments. This notion of a 'common mechanism' across therapies is supported by the fact that, despite a marked growth in treatment choice over the past 30 years, there have been no discernible additional clinical improvements [8]. The same broad clinical effects from different treatments for depressed young people are revealed in the UK IMPACT and ADAPT trials, which showed equivalent clinical outcomes from distinct therapies [2, 9]. So for depressed adolescents, whatever effective treatment they received, the rate and pace of recovery were broadly the same, as was the overall outcome.

From these findings we conjecture a strong likelihood of there being a common mechanism, present for all conversational treatments, with depressed adolescents.

Interestingly, almost all RCT studies also support a lower than expected pre-planned psychotherapy dose for a quicker than planned mental state and functional response. For example in the IMPACT study, although no more than 50% of the pre-planned interventions of any treatment had been delivered by 12 weeks, this 'dose' was associated with three-quarters of the total response achieved by end of treatment.

Finally, and of value for clinical theory and practice, is the finding that improvement continues for the 12 months post treatment: there was approximately a further 17% improvement in reduced depression symptoms and increased functioning with no further psychosocial or medication interventions.

We conjecture that the common mechanism(s) is activated early in treatment and accounts for the larger part of improvement occurring in the first 12 to 20 weeks or so of conversational treatment.

The IMPACT results across all treatments are summarised in Figure 4.5 below.

We hypothesise that a faster rate of change in the first phase of treatment is due to information gain about mental states and how they are experienced. We speculate that this is best achieved when they are provided by the therapist within a collaborative working relationship with the adolescent.

We consider that all therapies can promote early rapid improvement through one or more common mechanisms. These are quickly activated through effective episodes of conversational therapy. Our preliminary thoughts, given the current absence of evidence, are that:

A persisting therapeutic effect is best achieved through a collaborative and communicative working relationship. This in turn acts as a substrate for trust in psychotherapy by increasing general mental self-knowledge and mental acuity for the adolescent.

Increasing mental acuity means sharpening the mind and thereby being more aware of one's own mental processing, being ready to then effortfully make changes (getting started/activated) from a maladjusted to an adjusted mental state.

We consider that in the normal well-functioning adolescent mental state, information continuously enters the current mental state (CMS) via the sensory input system (eyes, ears, smell, touch, taste). The well-functioning current mental state, automatically and with little effort, processes all of this and ensures efficient, effective throughput of life experiences and their associated mental components. This theoretical framework is shown in Figure 4.6.

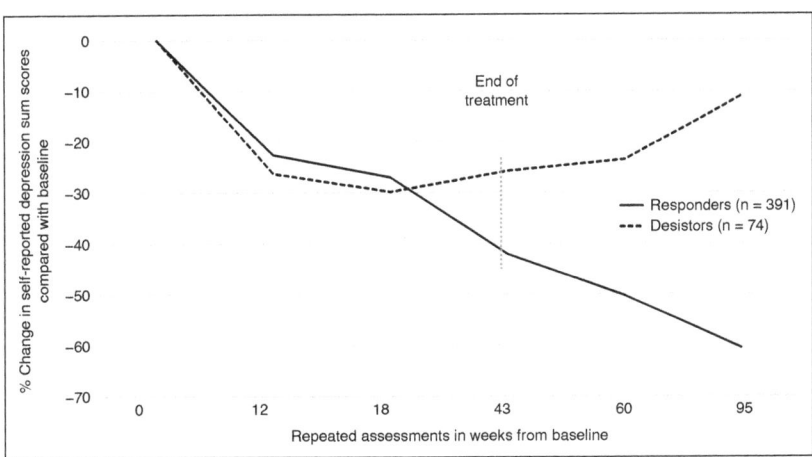

Figure 4.5 Percentage change in self-reported sum scores in depressed adolescents (n = 465)

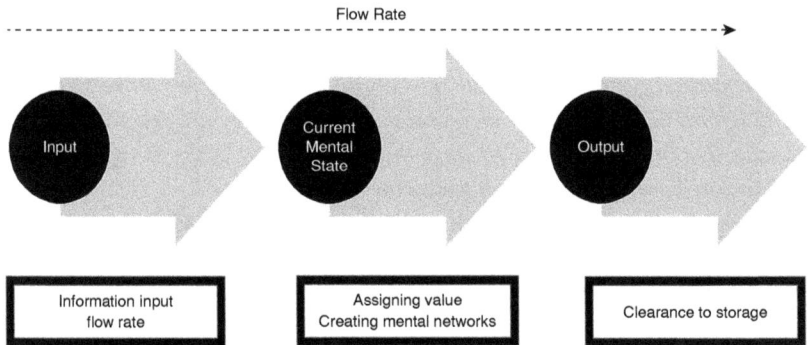

Figure 4.6 Information processing through current mental state (CMS)

Mental Components As a Network

Clinical discussion about current mental states will include the probable interactions of mental components that apparently connect to each other during mental illness in ways that they likely do not when mentally well [10]. For example poor sleeping and loss of energy may be logically considered as clinically interacting in undesirable ways during an episode of mental illness. These conversations about mind and body elements are part of the psychoeducation approach to understanding mental states that we use in BPI. Interestingly, these clinical discussions resonate with the increasing evidence that there are more interactions between mental components than previously considered. Researchers using (mathematically informed) network analytics have suggested, from a number of studies of depressed and anxious adults, that mental illnesses are actually a consequence of atypical psychopathological interactions between mental components: networks of illness [10]. The classical descriptive typologies of mental illnesses use counts, duration and severity of symptoms as diagnostic criteria but do not consider mental components as dynamically interacting networks or possible 'causes' of mental illness.

There appear to be many potentially clinically interesting aspects of such networks. One is the different strengths at which items may be interacting with each other. A network that has low numbers of significant interactions is known as a 'sparse network', which suggests a high degree of functionality and flexibility in the mind. In other words:

Low (network) interactions between components in a current mental state may imply healthy mental processing and a mental state capable of responding to experiences from the incoming environment in a flexible, adaptive, healthy manner.

In contrast, a 'dense network' contains many more interactions between mental components and is associated with less functionality and flexibility.

Compared with well adolescents, we conjecture that mentally unwell adolescents have a more densely connected mental network.

Density may also occur between some mental components, but not all. This may mean that overall density is not markedly different between well and unwell adolescents. Instead there may be a particular interaction or set of interactions that denotes increases in what is known as local density. The BPI clinician may perceive this in rigidity of thinking, difficulty solving life challenges, overthinking or similar constellations of everyday clinical presentation.

We know very little about the interactions, their impacts and origins, between symptoms in adolescents with mental health problems. This makes the value of network analytics unproven at this time when trying to explain therapeutic mechanisms. Within the IMPACT study, a preliminary exploration of the network characteristics of just depressive symptom interactions suggested there was indeed no overall difference in general global density from the beginning to the end of the study and therefore no effect of therapy on this measure [11]. There was, however, a denser local interaction between concentration and agitation in those who may have a less good treatment response [11]. These are highly preliminary observations.

Overall, we conjecture that future research might consider that:

Increased interactions between selected symptoms not usually closely connected in the current mental state may identify a psychopathological process that indexes and flags differences in treatment sensitivity.

Clearing the Current Mental State

A common experience in clinical assessment is to have an anxious and depressed young person saying 'I cannot stop thinking about my problems', 'I cannot get these thoughts out of my head' and 'Why do I feel so down all the time?' Such unwell young people are unable to distract themselves from their very difficult moods and thoughts and they become preoccupied and sometimes ruminative, turning the same components over and over in their minds. These preoccupying processes are the severe end of a continuum we all engage in when faced with a difficult experience or undesirable task we need to undertake. Under such conditions we may decide to focus on something else for a while or go for a walk to 'clear the mind'.

In treatment studies of depressed adolescents, preoccupying and brooding levels of thinking decline with psychological and pharmacological treatments in the same manner as depressive symptoms [2, 9, 12]. The evidence suggests treatment is as good at clearing ruminating mental processes from the current mental state as it is at reducing mental symptoms.

As we note in Figure 4.6 above, clearing the mind of recent adverse experiences and their associated mental components is a key task in keeping the mind efficient and processing incoming information from the environment. Without clearance we see that the current mental state gets rather static and cluttered such that incoming information likely cannot be processed very well.

We propose that a brooding and preoccupying mental response to incoming events and difficulties indicates a failure to maintain efficient clearance of information from the current mental state.

Summary

Overall, we have outlined the scientific case for BPI but also noted that diverse psychotherapies work with equal effectiveness for depressed adolescents. The changes in a range of depressive and non-depressive symptoms and functions found across all RCTs of depression in young people clearly show that all treatments are transdiagnostic: this is good for adolescents with emotional disorders where the presenting clinical features are almost always, indeed, comorbid and heterogeneous.

We remain unclear why or how psychotherapy works for young people with mental health problems. Here we have conjectured that BPI, which has low use of cognitive and psychoanalytic strategies, operates through three elements: information processing, network formation and subsequent clearance of the current mental state. We consider it more likely than not that BPI exerts its effects through general common mechanisms activated early in treatment that improve mental self-knowledge and mental acuity. This leads to a better understanding of the young person's own mental states. It is likely that utilising external, prosocial and physical actions helps improve mentalising, which in turn is likely to enhance clearance and reduce brooding and preoccupying psychopathology.

This theoretical framework is very much a 'work in progress' and remains to be tested and validated through further research and clinical practice.

REFERENCES

1. Goodyer I, Dubicka B, Wilkinson P, Kelvin R, Roberts C, Byford S et al. Selective serotonin reuptake inhibitors (SSRIs) and routine specialist care with and without cognitive behaviour therapy in adolescents with major depression: randomised controlled trial. *BMJ*. 2007;335(7611):142.

2. Goodyer IM, Reynolds S, Barrett B, Byford S, Dubicka B, Hill J et al. Cognitive-behavioural therapy and short-term psychoanalytic psychotherapy versus brief psychosocial intervention in adolescents with unipolar major depression (IMPACT): a multicentre, pragmatic, observer-blind, randomised controlled trial. *Health Technol Assess*. 2017;21(12):1–94.

3. Goodyer IM, Reynolds S, Barrett B, Byford S, Dubicka B, Hill J et al. Cognitive behavioural therapy and short-term psychoanalytical psychotherapy versus a brief psychosocial intervention in adolescents with unipolar major depressive disorder (IMPACT): a multicentre, pragmatic, observer-blind, randomised controlled superiority trial. *Lancet Psychiatry*. 2017;4(2):109–19.

4. Davies SE, Neufeld SAS, van Sprang E, Schweren L, Keivit R, Fonagy P et al. Trajectories of depression symptom change during and following treatment in adolescents with unipolar major depression. *J Child Psychol Psychiatry*. 2020;61(5):565–74.

5. O'Keeffe S, Martin P, Goodyer IM, Kelvin R, Dubicka B, IMPACT consortium et al. Prognostic implications for adolescents with depression who drop out of psychological treatment during a randomized controlled trial. *J Am Acad Child Adolesc Psychiatry*. 2019;58(10):983–92.

6. Midgley N, Hayes J, Cooper M, editors. *Essential Research Findings in Child and Adolescent Counselling and Psychotherapy*. London: Sage; 2017.

7. Weisz JR, Kuppens S, Ng MY, Eckshtain D, Ugueto AM, Vaughn-Coaxum R et al. What five decades of research tells us about the effects of youth psychological therapy: a multilevel meta-analysis and implications for science and practice. *Am Psychol*. 2017;72(2):79–117.

8. Eckshtain D, Kuppens S, Ugueto A, Ng MY, Vaughn-Coaxum R, Corteselli K et al. Meta-analysis: 13-year follow-up of psychotherapy effects on youth depression. *J Am Acad Child Adolesc Psychiatry*. 2020;59(1):45–63.

9. Goodyer IM, Dubicka B, Wilkinson P, Kelvin R, Roberts C, Byford S et al. A randomised controlled trial of cognitive behaviour therapy in adolescents with major depression treated by selective serotonin reuptake inhibitors: the ADAPT trial. *Health Technol Assess*. 2008;12(14):iii–iv, ix–60.

10. Borsboom D. A network theory of mental disorders. *World Psychiatry.* 2017;16(1):5–13.

11. Schweren L, van Borkulo CD, Fried E, Goodyer IM. Assessment of symptom network density as a prognostic marker of treatment response in adolescent depression. *JAMA Psychiatry.* 2018;75(1):98–100.

12. March J, Silva S, Petrycki S, Curry J, Wells K, Fairbank J et al. Fluoxetine, cognitive-behavioral therapy, and their combination for adolescents with depression: Treatment for Adolescents With Depression Study (TADS) randomized controlled trial. *JAMA.* 2004;292(7):807–20.

5 Practice Framework and Clinical Principles

This chapter describes the clinical methods that most likely make the best use of the clinical tools described in Chapters 3 and 6. First, we describe the three BPI domains of psychoeducation, social and personal prescribing and habilitation that constitute the framework of BPI.

Psychoeducation

Psychoeducation (PE) was originally defined as an information-giving strategy with systematic, structured and didactic knowledge transfer from the therapist to the recipient. The popularisation and development of the term psychoeducation began in the context of severe adult mental illness of schizophrenia. The primary purpose was educating relatives about the illness to aid ongoing management of the patient as well as supporting each other. The term widened to include helping patients directly to learn emotional and social skills as part of behavioural methods for treating more common mental illnesses in adults.

In BPI for adolescents, we have developed the notion of psychoeducation further to be an active and collaborative sharing process through which we convey an understanding, tuned and personally adapted to the young person and/or their parents, carers, teachers, etc., of the mental state and the nature and characteristics of the mental illness, such as depression, and offer strategies for intervention and recovery. Psychoeducation in BPI is not therefore an adjunct to treatment but a *key component* of the intervention. In BPI psychoeducation is active, enabling young patients to directly recover their normal mental state through the efforts of the therapist and themselves and to assist in engaging in adaptive prosocial and personal behaviours.

As noted in Chapter 3, we conceptualise psychoeducation as occurring through an open exchange of information whereby the adolescent offers information that contributes to the therapist's understanding of their (the adolescent's) mental state and life experiences. In return the therapist provides new knowledge so that there is a better understanding of mental states and their associations with behaviour. With BPI psychoeducation both the therapist and the adolescent are operating as a learner and a recipient of information: the therapist cannot provide the best pedagogic advice and explanation if they have not learned about the young person, how they view their experiences and what they have so far understood about their mental state.

Social and Personal Prescribing

Social prescribing in BPI shares some principles with the NHS England recommendations for social prescribing (www.england.nhs.uk/personalisedcare/social-prescribing). Social prescribing in BPI is achieved through shared planning and decision-making regarding what the adolescent will be doing in the social environment, to assist them in reducing mental health difficulties and increasing well-being. Unlike social prescribing principles for adults, this is not aimed at personalised budgets or legal rights to choose. We do consider that it is critically important that the adolescent patient perceives that they have selected social expereinces which are collaboratively agreed upon and likely to make a positive difference to their well-being through prosocial activity. Recent research has noted the value of the adolescent's social network as a key component in the building of resilience to future adversities and therefore in evolving adaptive mental states at times of adversity [1]. There is also evidence for the effectiveness of prosocial peer group and family activities in reducing subsequent mental health difficulties and decreasing the mental health risks associated with earlier childhood adversities [2].

The strategies may operate in a number of key social environments likely to include: (i) peer group and/or family relationships, (ii) school relations including those with teachers and other staff, (iii) the local neighbourhood, evaluating influences that may exist (good or bad) in the built environment such as parks, other open spaces, shops and leisure centres, (iv) the Internet and social media. The objective for the BPI therapist is to gain jointly agreed actions and exposure to the social world that will positively reorganise perceptions of environmental difficulties and associated personal performance. The focus can be education outcomes, developing or returning to hobbies, reactivating or learning personal interests and, critically, finding or returning to a habilitative place with others in the social world.

There is a strong focus on ensuring or re-engaging in social relations with peers, siblings, groups and teams. Family communication and relations may be a focus that closes any psychosocial gaps between the patient and their parents, grandparents and siblings. As noted, it is important to evaluate social exposure to the built environment and/or open spaces and this should be reviewed with the patient as it may be of relevance to any loss of social connectivity with or without others.

In addition, social prescribing must review the moderating effects of social media, including how the adolescent is using the Internet and what they are engaged with in this electronic social space. The same importance must be attached to how mobile phones and other electronic devices are used to engage with the more immediate social world and the extent to which these are impacting on well-being for better or worse.

Finally social prescribing should include behaviours aimed at personal achievements in the real world such as educational performance and the development of hobbies, pastimes and activities. These individual outputs generate value for the young person but also indirectly are likely to have social currency for others. This means that personal education, activities and individual development are all key component domains for social prescribing within BPI.

Habilitation

The third principle of BPI is for the therapist to be habilitative with the adolescent throughout the intervention. This is especially important as improvements become apparent in the mental state and behaviour. Habilitation means 'to make suitable or fit' and is a conversational process aimed at helping individuals to attain, keep or improve skills and functioning for daily living. We see habilitation as an important concept in mentally ill adolescents who are developing an understanding of themselves and the world, expanding their social experiences and communicating in new ways with peers. It includes learning skills in personal, educational and family settings. We see mental illness in this age range as disrupting the act or process of 'becoming fit' or of 'making fit' for a particular purpose: that is, mental illness is preventing the habilitation of experiences for personal growth and development. Mental illness can impair participation and performance in one or more environments and BPI therapists have a key role in collaboratively advising and supporting adolescents as they reduce the negative impact of mental illnesses such as depression.

Of course there is likely to be the need for some rehabilitation as well, since mentally ill adolescents will also be regaining and reusing skills, abilities or knowledge that may have been compromised as a result of a mental illness.

The terms habilitation and rehabilitation have been of considerable value in the field of disability, being seen as processes that seek to attain maximum independence, full physical, mental, social and vocational ability, and full inclusion and participation in all aspects of life. We consider that these health and well-being principles are applicable to the mentally ill young person suffering with a mental illness that is preventing the learning of new mental and behavioural skills and disabling those already attained.

Clinical Practice Principles

Here we briefly describe the key aspects of the therapy processes as a prelude to Chapters 6 and 7, which provide working details of the BPI clinical method.

Getting to Know You

We have emphasised the development of a working collaborative relationship between the BPI therapist and the adolescent. This is best achieved through an active 'getting to know you' conversational approach. Here the therapist takes the lead in the opening 15 minutes of the first session to explore and understand as comprehensively as possible the adolescent's social environment. This includes the structure, perception and experience of family, friends, the built environment, school and personal interests, hobbies and habits.

In BPI this is the first task before turning to a detailed discussion of presenting problems and current mental state. Getting to know you is about setting a social picture of the young person's social contexts so that the three strands of BPI (psychoeducation, social prescribing and habilitation) can be woven together through the use of the tools outlined in Chapters 3 and 6. This active induction of personal conversation is a therapist task but where adolescents wish to express opinions and ask questions then those aspects should be followed and discussed. The extent to which the therapist reveals aspects of themselves is not clear-cut in any therapy. Here we would encourage BPI therapists to share like-minded interests and similar hobbies or activities. For example, adolescents may reveal they are very fond of the family dog and the therapist may declare they like dogs and have one at home. This 'pet conversation' can include showing pictures of family pets and enquiring about names and how they were given them. Revealing therapist aspects is, however, led by the social history and context reported by the adolescents, not the other way round, and must of course remain within safeguarding and good governance rules. It is unhelpful for the therapist to introduce social themes of no clear-cut meaning to the young person.

This collation of social context is woven into an understanding of where the young person believes themselves to be right now. This includes the problems they are faced with, the factors that they perceive as being responsible for the current difficulties, their current mental and physical state that may be a result of these problems and the impact all this has had on their current function. At the end of this section of the first therapy session there should be a clear summation in the mind of the BPI therapist about the young person's current social environment and context, their social network, personal interests, presenting problems, current mental state and the impact of these on their behaviour and personal function.

Keeping You Safe

Brief Psychosocial Intervention therapists have a responsibility to keep young people safe during therapy. Clinical interviewing and therapy methods necessarily involve assessing risk to safety. Risks may come from the external environment or from an abnormal mental state. Adolescents can be 'at risk' because of harms and hazards than may accrue from their social context such as assault or maltreatment, deviant group pressures to commit offences and to use hazardous substances. Importantly, the adolescent's abnormal mental state may create risks through desires to self-harm or suicidal thoughts and actions. These are critically important to assess and understand; therapists should seek supervision and support for themselves when such risks are revealed. No BPI should be practised without access to professional support and ongoing supervision. The origins of these risks may be in the immediate social context, social media or within the adolescent themselves. When the therapist and the adolescent agree there is a risk to the safety of the young person then the therapist must implement a safety plan and ensure that this is in place and can be activated when required. Details are covered in the next chapter, which outlines the clinical manual guiding BPI therapy practice.

What Matters to You

As we noted in 'Getting to Know You', it is important to understand what matters to the young person. These include:

- me (hobbies/fun, physical health, looking after myself)
- the things that matter to me (education/work, things I need to do, the bigger picture)
- the people that matter to me (family, friends, boyfriend/girlfriend).

Monitoring and evaluating these aspects of behaviour are very important for intervention decision-making. There may be a clear need to discuss, clarify and intervene when the things that matter are considered deleterious to mental health and well-being.

Healthy Habits

Brief psychosocial intervention emphasises the importance of well-being strategies and the promotion of healthy habits. Physical fitness, sleep hygiene, eating sensibly, digital life, smoking, alcohol misuse and illicit drug use are all topics that should be part of the collaborative dialogue. The adolescent may need facts and figures and is certainly likely to want advice and strategies to improve one or more of these features.

Doing More of What Matters to You

Habilitation and rehabilitation strategies should be employed to revisit, re-emphasise and support the activities and social behaviours that matter to the young person. It is not advisable to accept a single instance of social success, such as making new friends or re-engaging with old ones. Brief psychosocial intervention therapists should ensure as much as possible that prosocial behaviours are more than a one-off experience and that improvements in the current mental state are maintained as treatment proceeds.

Dealing with Difficulties and Keeping Things Going

Therapy is effortful and a key role for the therapist is to ensure that the difficulties and efforts that are likely to accrue to gain mental health improvements are managed effectively. Therapists must remember to check on how difficult mental and behavioural gains have been. This can include acknowledging the effort required to improve in mind and behaviour, supporting the maintenance of such gains and encouraging further positive experiences. New difficulties may also occur during treatment and it is important to evaluate such life events and help where possible to reduce any threats these may pose to clinical progress. Personally disappointing life events during treatment may prolong the time to recovery, perhaps through creating uncertainty in the young person regarding whether their progress is real or can be sustained. At these times the therapist must actively support progress, argue strongly against self-doubt and continue to encourage and support progress made and progress to come.

Getting Help from Others

If the young person's social network/system is needed to deliver therapy strategies, BPI therapists will facilitate this. This may be when social plans require help to be achieved. Sometimes the young person might need help completing activities. It might be a lift to the cinema to watch a film with friends, a hand getting some sports equipment from the loft or help from a teacher to finish a tricky piece of coursework. BPI therapists must monitor the need for getting help from others and consider why it is judged necessary, see that this occurs and so enable the best opportunity for therapeutic effectiveness.

Planning for the Future and Ending Well

We believe that ending therapy should be thought about early in treatment. Because BPI is designed and practised as brief therapy, it is not expected that patients will be in treatment beyond 6 months. Indeed, what we know from the research projects is that the usual duration for BPI is between 6 and 18 weeks receiving between 4 to 11 sessions (median = 6). So towards the end, agreed through the working collaboration with the young person, it is important for the BPI therapist to review the gains made during therapy and discuss how these can be maintained and built on. How is the young person going to continue moving forwards, increasing their social skills, personal performance and educational objectives? Has the adolescent been sensitised to recognise warning signals in the environment and in themselves that they may again be at risk of mental difficulties? If so, what are the strategies that they know will reduce the risk, improve protection and resilience, and enhance well-being? These latter points emphasise the importance of the habilitative learning that should have occurred through BPI active and collaborative psychoeducation and prosocial strategies with the therapist.

In the next chapter we provide a workbook-style description of clinical practice and principles with some illustrative clinical examples of the techniques.

REFERENCES

1. Fritz J, Stochl J, Goodyer IM, van Harmelen AL, Wilkinson PO. Embracing the positive: an examination of how well resilience factors at age 14 can predict distress at age 17. *Transl Psychiatry*. 2020;10(1):272.
2. Askelund AD, Schweizer S, Goodyer IM, van Harmelen AL. Positive memory specificity is associated with reduced vulnerability to depression. *Nat Hum Behav*. 2019;3(3):265–73.

6   Clinical Styles and Therapy Tools

BPI Core Components of Intervention

To recap, there are three key practice principles of BPI:

(i)   pedagogic psychoeducation: understanding mental states
(ii) social and personal prescribing: the environment as intervention
(iii) habilitation: supporting new learning and prosociality.

These are the domains in which the tools of practice are used to achieve and maintain recovery, defined as good mental health and well-being. Here we describe the method of engagement used in BPI and subsequently we expand on a set of conversational tools that can be selected and used to achieve the objectives of improved understanding of mental health, being prosocial and active in the environment and remembering to use mental health skills that support the maintenance of well-being during and after therapy. Recall that in Chapter 4 we noted that improvement continues for a year after therapy ends, which we suggest is habilitation underpinning continued recovery.

Establishing a Collaborative Relationship

Conversational treatments all require establishing therapeutic collaboration between the therapist and young person to achieve the agreed goals through therapy. This collaborative framework is developed in the first session and remains in place throughout the length of the intervention. With young people this is best achieved by adolescents being actively involved in determining how to proceed, ideally with their parents, if available. It is probably helpful to provide an information sheet to the family about the aims and purposes of the intervention prior to the first session. The type of collaboration most suitable for brief psychotherapy is what we have called an 'open exchange collaborative model'. In this model we assume that the most efficient and effective way to gain an alliance with the adolescent is for the therapist to be active, engaging and informative. Open exchange collaborative processing should therefore begin with the therapist asking if the adolescent has an understanding and expectation of meeting with them. It is important to appreciate the expectations that the adolescent brings to the meeting. The therapist should ask if they know who they are meeting with, if they were aware they had been referred and what the aims and purposes of the therapy are. In practical terms this means that the therapist will ask questions about the adolescent's personal experiences in an information-gathering manner which shows interest and inquiry about their lives. In return the therapist should be willing and able to provide an educative discourse about the young person's mental illness, giving a hypothesised explanation for their distress and difficulties. Using an open exchange collaborative framework, the therapist should also say something about their professional self and describe the principles of BPI being used to help with their problems.

For example, a first session exchange may reveal that the adolescent really did not want to come and talk to a stranger about their problems, and it was their parent's idea; the therapist in return might say they were sorry to hear that but in their experience most teens with problems do find it a good thing to talk with a mental health specialist. This can be followed up with a clear statement that the therapy is for and about the young person and is best achieved by working together. This is an example of open exchange, which should be utilised throughout the intervention. We consider that the open exchange methodology facilitates the practice of BPI and we conjecture that it promotes the low dose–high response effects that we see with psychotherapies of quite different theoretical backgrounds and intervention styles, as we described in Chapter 4. The principles underpinning an open exchange collaboration with an adolescent are shown in Figure 6.1.

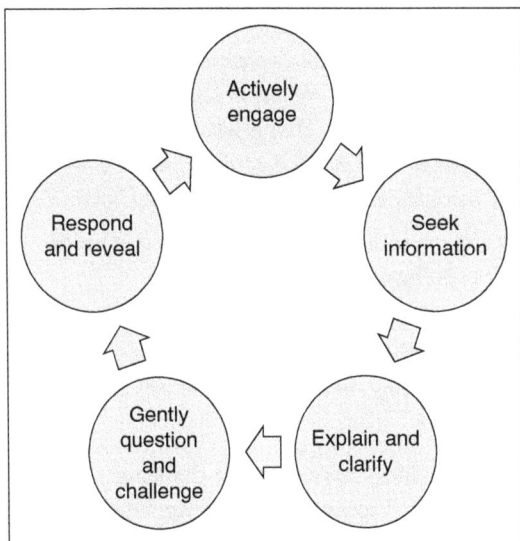

Figure 6.1 Open exchange collaboration

The figure shows that an open exchange collaboration builds a therapeutic alliance with the young person through actively enquiring from the outset about themselves and their experiences. The therapist should be willing to take the initiative in these discussions and not accept silences, which can be uncomfortable for both and are non-productive: no information-gathering and no setting up of a collaborative relationship. The adolescent is encouraged and supported openly to begin their story, describing themselves as a person, their social context and their lived experiences as well as their understanding of their difficulties. Adolescents may not have shared some of their own musings, thoughts and reflections on their experiences or mental state and this can be recognised by the therapist, for example:

> **Therapist**: *Thanks for telling me about your family members and how you are getting on at school and the recent difficulties that have been a real trouble to you. I wanted to ask you about these a bit more, starting with what is going on in your mind about the troubles you have talked about. What's it like for you right now in there? Describe your moods and thoughts and feelings as they are right now if you can.*
>
> **Young person**: *(hesitates, averts gaze and looks uncomfortable)*
>
> **Therapist**: *I know it is unusual to be asked about your moods and thoughts but that's a big part of what you and I are trying to get to grips with together so we can figure out what's best for you right now. Let me explain that we all have moods, thoughts and feelings that change as we have experiences. We get on with our lives, don't we, even when we are a bit sad or gloomy, even grumpy and irritable, but these moods pass, don't they? That's normal for all of us. What is happening to you right now seems as though your mind has not been able to get on with life. That is what we need to understand and to do that you need to help me by describing what I call your 'mental state': the moods, thoughts and feelings you currently have.*
>
> **Young Person**: *(hesitant) But I've never done this before. It's kind of weird and I don't like some of the things going on in my head.*
>
> **Therapist**: *I know but it is going to be less weird when you tell me and together we figure out what it's like in there for you and what we need to do about it. Sometimes the mind has things in it that are a bit weird, even scary, but let us see what it is together.*

As illustrated above, the therapist uses questions and gentle challenge to clarify uncertainties and ambiguities in the adolescent's story. The vignette indicates the value of active engagement through open exchange about experiences and current mental state as a component of building a collaborative relationship with the young person.

Therapist Styles for BPI

A BPI therapist has to consider taking a stance towards the depressed and anxious adolescent that may be somewhat different to practice with adults or younger children. The vignette above illustrates that the therapist may need to utilise a degree of challenge to activate collaboration. This must be done with a clear explanation of what the benefit is to the adolescent of engaging with the therapist in an open and clear exchange of information. These principles of conversational style are outlined in Figure 6.2.

The therapist style is aimed at forming an alliance with the adolescent that should last throughout the therapy. Alliance is where two parties agree on a common goal and how this should be achieved. This can only realistically occur through the collaborative relationship being built from the first session. An alliance through collaboration is an arrangement between therapist and adolescent to share information and knowledge to produce a formulation and treatment plan that fits the needs of the young person. Fundamental to successful alliance formation is the therapist being an active 'alliance and educative partner', offering encouragement through a pedagogic-educative stance towards mental health problems and associated behavioural difficulties. Information-gathering

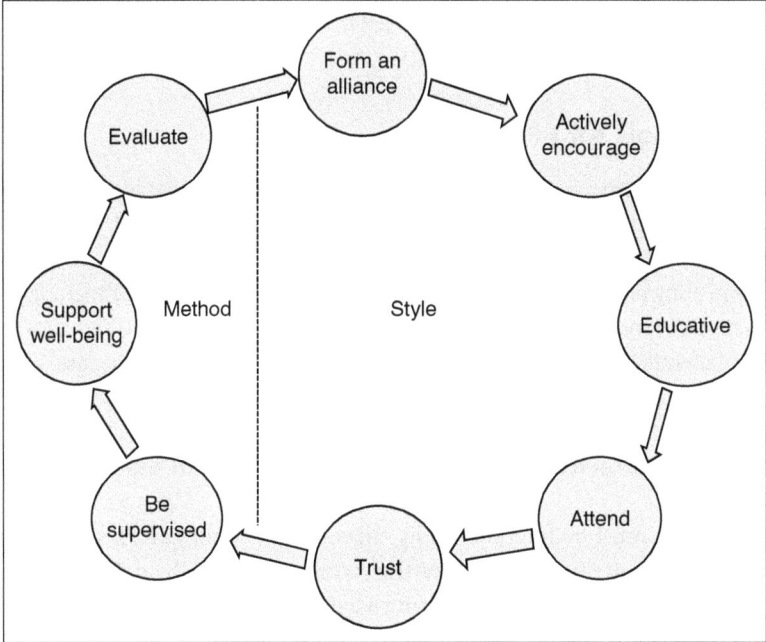

Figure 6.2 BPI therapist style and clinical method

and sharing, clarifying ambiguities and meaning with the adolescent, hearing their understanding of experiences that are important to them and appreciating the contexts within which they have been exposed to life events are critical elements in therapist techniques to elicit a formulation and consider interventions going forward.

This approach is a continuation of the active collaborating style, which means that through treatment the therapist is not allowing the adolescent to sit in the clinic room brooding, preoccupied or worried but is actively eliciting their thoughts and feelings. Active therapy is asking directly: How are you right now? What are you thinking about? Do you feel as you usually do and, if not, can you please describe 'your current feeling state'?

This active style is likely to engage adolescents rapidly and generate the trust needed to further develop this collaborative engagement. The therapist must ensure that they attend to what is being reported and that the formulation is created with a full appreciation of the personal experience of the adolescent, the contexts within which lived experiences happened and the information-gathering that is necessary to formulate a treatment plan in the best interests of the young person.

Figure 6.2 also shows three method components showing that BPI therapists should not work alone and should be supervised and preferably work in a clinical environment that is multidisciplinary and supports an evidence-based approach to intervention.

Therapist Tools for BPI

We believe that the therapist style and method described above lead to interventions that can be achieved using one or more conversational strategies selected from a suite of such 'talking tools'. There is no single therapy strategy for a given clinical diagnostic group. As such, it is important that BPI therapists have a clinical toolkit from which they can select the conversational approach likely to generate the greatest clinical effectiveness for each individual case. The BPI toolkit currently in use is shown in Figure 6.3.

Interpersonal Effectiveness and Fostering a Culture of Being Able to Help

A BPI therapist must be interpersonally effective and communicate clearly to attain the most desirable outcomes for the young person. With adolescents we consider this is best achieved by adopting a balanced, optimistic stance, which is characterised by being confident and using friendly, encouraging dialogue. Establishing a culture of being able to help facilitates the tool of interpersonal

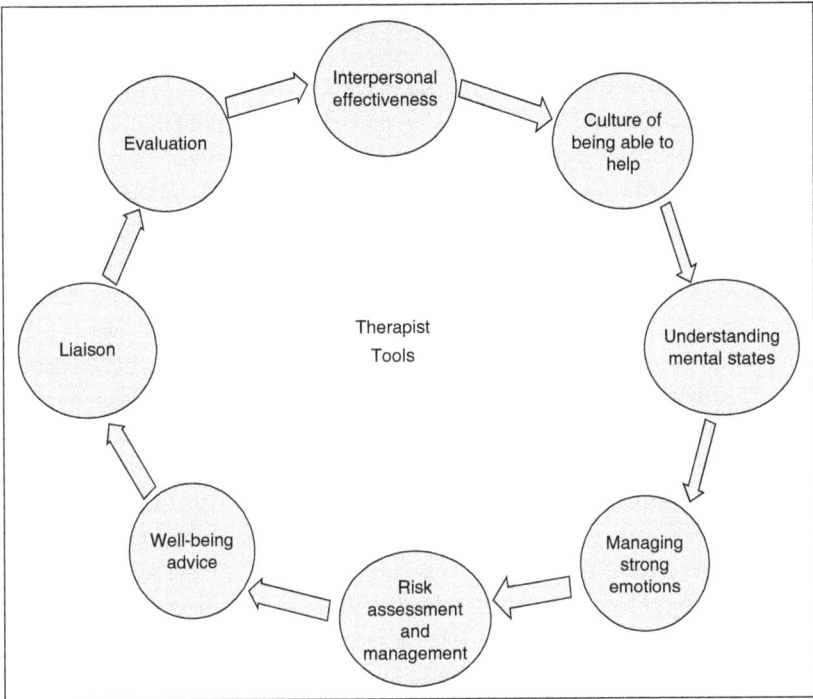

Figure 6.3 BPI therapist toolkit

effectiveness. These tools foster alliance formation through active collaboration as a prelude to designing, with the adolescent, bespoke social and personal interventions. We consider that, compared with a non-relating or overly didactic style, an active, friendly and encouraging therapist is more likely to help a mentally unwell adolescent discard their current mental illness in favour of a return to a more adaptive mental state and thereby well-being. This positive therapeutic stance is well recognised as important for psychological treatments at most stages in the life cycle. During adolescence, however, the style of alliance formation and encouraging a positive approach to mental and behavioural difficulties using a friendly open style may have a key early role in treatment adherence [1]. In contrast, not achieving a positive therapeutic stance by the second session is likely to be associated with non-attendance for further psychological treatment [2, 3].

Understanding Mental States

In BPI, it is assumed that adolescents have yet to develop sufficient mastery and control of their mental activity and can be aided by a psychoeducative approach. Brief psychosocial intervention has a pedagogic principle in therapy and assumes that imparting knowledge about and creating a better understanding of mental states is in itself therapeutic. This pedagogic approach aids a young person in understanding how their current mental state (CMS) is working and helps them to monitor mentalising (i.e. what their mind is doing). By providing knowledge about how the current mental state is affecting them, we are informing and helping the adolescent to learn (habilitate) about what happens to moods, thoughts, feelings and behaviours when mentalising is going wrong.

Perhaps the first of the psychoeducative objectives is informing the adolescent in a conversational and collaborative manner that their current mental state is an active, dynamic, mentalising processor that is constantly open to the continuous flow of information coming in via their senses from the environment. The therapist outlines to the adolescent that their CMS is malfunctioning and not working in its owner's best interests. Psychoeducation also needs to inform the adolescent that mentalising is effortful. This includes the purpose of assigning personal meaning to the incoming experience, the value or importance of which may be changed or moderated by prior experiences. The BPI therapist discusses with the adolescent the real possibility that when we have mental health problems, we cannot always trust our own judgements and decisions made during this time. This is because an abnormal mental state is prone to creating errors in perception, appraisal, personal meaning- and decision-making of incoming experience. Psychoeducative strategies will suggest that following the advice 'inside your head' and acting on it may not always be in your best interests if you are mentally unwell. The BPI therapist will find these potentially complex discussions about understanding mental states and what happens when they go wrong are facilitated by adopting the positive therapeutic stance described above and maintaining a balanced and optimistic culture of being able to help.

Appreciating the Abnormal Mental State

From the illness perspective we contend that the adolescent will benefit from an explanation of the dynamic importance of the current mental state. Engaging in a dialogue with the young person (*tools and techniques: information exchange component using effective communication and an active pedagogic style*) and providing a description of how mental components can interact with each other are further contributions to strengthening an understanding of mental states. We can begin by considering the flow of mental components and experiences through the mind and their effect on the relations of mental components with each other. We suggest that a slowed mental state is a characteristic of an inefficient internal environment where mental components (i.e. moods, thoughts, feelings, sensations) are no longer flowing through the mind at an optimal rate. A suboptimal flow rate sets the conditions for a more strongly associated set of mental items with each other in a way that produces a denser mental network and impedes the efficiency of clearing information from the mind. Consider a case illustration:

Jennifer was a 15-year-old with no prior mental illness in her or her family. She lived at home with her parents and younger sister. Jennifer had been referred as an urgent case by her family doctor, having recently become socially isolated, sleeping poorly and no longer talking with friends. Jennifer had offered no explanation for her change of behaviour and was withdrawn and silent with her family doctor until he asked if life was still worth living, when she shook her head.

The therapist took an active, gentle style in the first interview and enquired about Jennifer as a person with no direct mention of her mental state. Jennifer talked quite easily with the therapist and was able to say that she felt sad and rather empty, which was both strange and a little frightening as she did not know where these moods and thoughts had come from. She said she felt out of control of how her mind was working and yes, when asked directly by the therapist, she would like to 'get her mind back to be herself again!' The therapist said that the next time they met they would talk more about understanding her mind and how to figure out a way to get it back. The therapist was open, active and offered a culture of being able to help with confidence and a genuine smile.

At the second session, five working days later, the therapist asked Jennifer to describe her current mental state. Together they worked out the predominant current mood, thoughts and feelings/sensations (tools and techniques: collaborative alliance). *They also discussed if her mind was able to 'work' as it normally would. Jennifer said no and the therapist asked her to offer up some 'reasons' for this. The 'to and fro' discussion* (tools and techniques: information exchange in a working collaborative alliance within a culture of being able to help) *produced an agreement that Jennifer could not change things in her head as easily as usual. Her moods and thoughts were not her usual ones, things were jammed (her word) together, taking up all the 'space in her mind' and difficult to shift. Expending a great deal of effort to get back to normal had been to no avail. As a result, she had begun to be preoccupied and brooding over her loss of mentalising (therapist's word) and how mental components (therapist's word) were 'running into one another' (therapist's phrase that Jennifer agreed summed up her mind right now: her words for her mind were 'crowded' and 'sticky').*

The loss of optimal mental flow leading to inefficient mentalising increases the risk for secondary difficulties: for example, a greater degree of brooding and preoccupation, as noted in the clinical vignette. Further atypical mental consequences might include inattention to new information coming in from the environment as the mental state is occupied, with no clearance of the CMS to memory. We conjecture that it is therapeutic to impart a set of working mechanisms offering a comprehensive knowledge and understanding of why their mental state is currently inefficient compared with their normal processing.

Managing Strong Emotions

The word 'emotion' dates back to 1579, from the French word *émouvoir*, meaning 'to stir up'. It was not until the nineteenth century, however, that the word 'emotion' entered the common English language, covering all types of feeling states. The term 'emotion' is now generally considered as denoting a strong or intense feeling state. There is, however, currently no scientific consensus on the definition of an emotion. Here, for clinical purposes, we consider that emotions are psychological states brought on by neurophysiological activity. This means that brain changes evoke a subjective mental output as a feeling state along a continuum of pleasurable to non-pleasurable feelings.

In BPI we want to encourage adaptive emotions to dominate the mental state. Therefore a discussion and assessment of 'feelings' early in treatment is recommended. This should examine how feelings are represented in the mental state, gaining a shared understanding of the role they may play in determining action and what methods the young person uses to reduce intensity that may be contributing to overall impairment. Intensity is the force of a property, analogous to the brightness of a light, whereas severity is the overall negative effect of a property, for example reducing the ability to see when a light is excessively bright or dark.

The orientation of the assessment is that emotions, generally, organise and facilitate adaptive responses to environmental challenges. Emotions are therefore evoked by environmental input, contribute to mental state content and connectivity and influence the behavioural output. Emotions are therefore largely beneficial insofar as they inform and prepare individuals to respond to environmental challenges. They play a crucial role in organising social interactions and personal relationships.

From the clinical perspective emotional dysregulation may arise when exposed to an undesirable recent life event, leading to sudden and often unexpected intense emotions. In these circumstances, maladaptive feeling states can emerge (sadness, fear, irritability) and contribute to the emergence of a typical mental states and impairing behaviours. The BPI therapist is likely to be engaged in managing and reducing the intensity of such emotions to reduce overall mental dysregulation, with the objective of recovering an adaptive mental state and associated behaviour.

The BPI therapist needs to make clear to the adolescent what normal emotions and their purposes are as outlined above. Working collaboratively, they aim to reduce intensity from negative emotions (i.e. in sad, fearful or irritable states) and/or increase intensity for positive emotions (i.e. happiness, contentment) in the mental state and offer strategies to promote prosocial and personal behavioural actions that support this. Given the nature of consultations, some of this may occur during a session as emotions are triggered and displayed. Here 'pacing' of the discussion and supporting of the therapeutic alliance become key.

Risk Assessment and Management

Amongst adolescents with mood-related mental health problems, almost all have been exposed to one or more undesirable life events or ongoing difficulties in the preceding 12 months. These undesirable experiences not only increase the liability of mental health difficulties but may also reduce sensitivity to treatment. Adolescents may also engage in risk behaviours such as substance misuse, excess alcohol use or smoking and these personal habits may also impair treatment effects. Overall, in BPI the therapist should assess proximal risk factors both at the time of presentation and for the previous 3 months. This should include a full discussion of their potential influences on treatment response and general progress as part of the formulation. Of course, young people may also be exposed to events or experiences that reduce the liability of mental health difficulties or in theory increase treatment effects. Examples of social factors of these protective types include positive confiding and supportive family relationships, a peer group network that is accessible and active and engaging in personal hobbies. There is good evidence that improving social relationships with family and friends during adolescence reduces the mental health risk effects of prior childhood adversities. This may occur through creating positive memories from proximal social experiences that reduce the negative effects associated with the recall of difficult childhood experiences thereby fostering resilience in the adolescent [4]. The clinical implications of understanding the impact of risk and protective factors are related to treatment response: increasing environmental protective factors can reduce the negative effects of prior risks on the likelihood of treatment response. Protection contributes to the building of resilience processes, which reduce the liability to subsequent mental illnesses. Resilience is not a factor but a mental process emerging as a consequence of prosocial experiences with family, friends, school and community. BPI can contribute to resilience building through each of the three domains of psychoeducation, social prescribing and habilitation. Assessing risk and protection factors therefore guides the BPI therapist in terms of the intervention type but in particular emphasises the value of social prescribing in improving social relationships with important others in family, friends, school and community environments. This balance between risk and protection is shown in Figure 6.4.

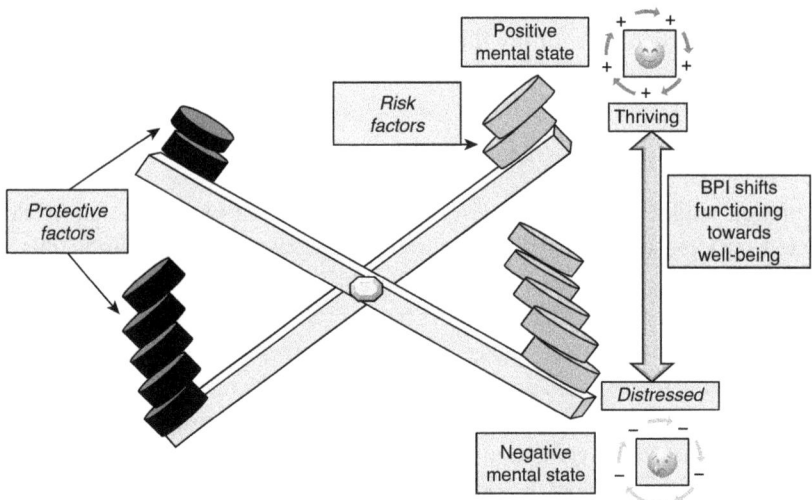

Figure 6.4 Therapeutic framework for risk and protective factors

As the figure shows, when the adolescent is loaded with more protective than risk factors there is a greater probability that there will be a positive and adaptive mental state. In contrast, when the balance is in favour of risk over protection factors there is an increased risk of a negative and maladaptive current mental state.

Assessing and discussing risk and protection provides explication and clarification of important environmental components of personal experience. This is because discussing these experiences with the adolescent and elucidating their meaning and impact are psychoeducative: clarifying misconceptions and misunderstandings about the experiences and how they have been considered by the young person can contribute to reducing brooding and preoccupation, decreasing worry and increasing positive feelings. For many mentally unwell adolescents, providing clarity about their difficult and perhaps perplexing risk environments and their implications for the future may be treatment itself. This psychoeducative strategy around environmental risk and protection redraws the implications of bad experiences in a different light and can instil hope and purpose for the future. We strongly encourage BPI therapists to undertake a careful risk/protection analysis early and certainly within the first three treatment sessions.

Promoting Healthy Habits and Well-Being

Healthy habits constitute a further domain of therapeutic tools within the BPI toolbox. Fostering a return to or adding new healthy habits also promotes well-being. The components of sleep, diet, substance use, digital life and physical exercise are the focus of collaborative discussions and planning for change, if required.

Sleep disruption in depressed adolescents is one of the most common presenting problems. Overall, sleep difficulties reduce substantially with treatment but in a few cases they do not and specific sleep hygiene intervention may be required [5]. Discussing and explaining that the poor-quality sleep being experienced is part of the current mental illness and will improve with the current treatment is, we believe, a valuable step in assisting with treatment compliance.

Reviewing nutrition with a currently depressed adolescent is an important assessment strategy. There is no clear-cut evidence that dietary factors alone can predict mental health problems or treatment response but there is some evidence to support the hypothesis that nutritional factors may influence mood in young people [6]. From the practice perspective we should work on the assumption that a balanced diet is a healthy habit that contributes to well-being. This is likely to become a topic for discussion in adolescents who show risky eating and dietary habits whilst presenting with mood-related mental health difficulties. Discussing eating habits gives the therapist an opportunity to describe the potential value of a balanced diet that includes vegetables, fruit and fish, and provide advice on being disciplined about lowering the intake of additives, chemically induced fats and high-carbohydrate foods.

Physical activity is another healthy habit to focus on in formulation and discussions about well-being. Of particular note is not the extent of moderate to vigorous activity undertaken by the adolescent but the amount of sedentary time undertaken. High sedentary behaviour over the adolescent years is associated with greater depressive symptoms by the end of adolescence [7]. Sedentary behaviour can also be associated with increased screen time, which itself may be associated with subsequent lower educational performance [8]. From the clinical perspective adolescents can be educated and supported to engage in persistent light activity such as walking and going up and down stairs. Potential resistance to such activity occurs when adolescents are encouraged to undertake moderate to severe exercise as a goal, which has no additional benefits for mental well-being over light exercise. There is also an association between food intake and physical activity both influencing mood and behaviour [9]. Therefore attention to increasing low-level activity is a valuable intervention for improving food intake, well-being and personal performance. The everyday interplay between food, exercise and well-being is an important educative component to get across in this maturing phase of the life-course.

Increasingly, mental health assessments and interventions need to consider the influence of social media. Here the role of collaborative relationships with the adolescent and their parents may be key: the therapist needs to elicit information about current use to evaluate and manage risk and may, in some cases, need to discuss and advise on boundary-setting to support safety online. This is a non-trivial matter as adolescents can find themselves drawn to an unhealthy, hazardous or abusive experience online.

Finally, discussions are necessary regarding the possible use of hazardous substances. The use of cannabinoids and related substances is dangerous for adolescents with current mental health problems and should be explained as such. The potential mental health risks of caffeine and stimulant drinks whilst suffering with mental health difficulties should also be underlined and an understanding of how, if at all, they are used by the adolescent.

Well-Being Advice

The final component is to give well-being advice, which involves embedding a key set of values within the adolescent for keeping well. There is currently no agreed definition of well-being but the concept of mental well-being in young people appears to be more than just the absence of disease [10]. Well-being can be seen as a resource that allows people to realise their aspirations, satisfy their needs and cope with the environment in order to live a long, productive and fruitful life. For many adolescents this well-being component is likely to be habilitative; that is, the BPI therapist will be using psychoeducation to impart well-being advice often for the first time. There should be an emphasis on encouraging and supporting prosocial experiences and personal achievements to confirm subjective wellness in the real world. This is likely to include important others in friendship and family groups confirming and reaffirming the value of the young person and their talents over time. The BPI therapist is therefore encouraging (habilitating) adolescents to learn the art of keeping well and being able to recognise and value the experience of well-being through being valued by others for who they are. This positivist approach is holistic such that the adolescent patient should be able to recognise a sense of happiness and contentment within themselves. Brief psychosocial intervention therapy should also help the adolescent learn and use the association between personal contentment and life satisfaction but this educative phase has to be mindful that young people, unlike adults, are maturing and concepts such as contentment and life satisfaction will likely change with age and environmental context.

Habilitation strategies in BPI are likely to emphasise the importance and value to well-being of developing personal as well as social interests, being pro-social with peers and supporting the demands of taking other people's views into consideration as well as their own. A second well-being strategy concerns enhancing mental awareness development and encouraging a preference for focusing on mental content that values the self and drives curiosity and partici-pation in the world around them.

In BPI the therapist helps the young person to favour well-being over mental illness, which is likely to include not paying attention to intrusive negative moods and thoughts about the self and others. The young person is helped to understand that such thoughts are atypical, may lead to increasing interactions with other mental components and increase the risk of mental illness. Combining that habili-tative experience with adaptive externalising behaviours such as avoiding social isolation and speaking with friends or family can degrade negative mindsets and improve a bias towards a positive mental state. These well-being promotion tactics can be clinically validated by setting goals that emphasise social connectedness and personal productivity in the home, school and neighbourhood environments.

Liaison

Like many methods in young people's mental health, BPI must be aware of and assess the need for liaising and collaborating with those in the wider social system. Involving parents, where possible and agreed, is part of the immediate treatment but be aware of the need to communicate with others where risk and protec-tive factors may emerge. The school and community environments may need to be liaised with directly, as might friends and siblings. Brief psychosocial inter-vention retains an open stance to social systems where the adolescents may be exposed to adverse experiences, and these may become domains for social inter-vention. Professional liaison, such as with primary health care workers/provid-ers and schoolteachers, may be an important source for validating information, including past medical history or current education and peer group difficulties.

Assessing liaison domains is a useful tool to enable the nature and charac-teristics of the social system that are within the scope of BPI social and psycho-educative strategies.

Evaluation

Finally, we recommend that progress with BPI is evaluated over the course of treatment. This is best achieved by measuring in parallel both therapist and adolescent (and, if feasible, parent/carer) perceptions of clinical progress.

The adolescent (and, if feasible, the parent/carer) can be asked to complete a self-report questionnaire at the first assessment and then at sequential points over the course of treatment, perhaps at monthly intervals. In addition, session-by-session 'outcomes' recordings can be made, although trends over time may fluctuate so it can be difficult to understand and use these immediate therapy measures. Clinicians can record their global view easily enough by noting worsening, no change or improvement in symptoms and behaviours.

REFERENCES

1. Dhanak D, Thackeray L, Dubicka B, Kelvin R, Goodyer IM, Midgley N. Adolescents' experiences of brief psychosocial intervention for depression: an interpretative phenomenological analysis of good-outcome cases. *Clin Child Psychol Psychiatry.* 2020;25(1):106–18.
2. O'Keeffe S, Martin P, Goodyer IM, Wilkinson P, IMPACT consortium, Midgley N. Predicting dropout in adolescents receiving therapy for depression. *Psychother Res.* 2018;28(5):708–21.
3. O'Keeffe S, Martin P, Goodyer IM, Kelvin R, Dubicka B, IMPACT consortium et al. Prognostic implications for adolescents with depression who drop out of psychological treatment during a randomized controlled trial. *J Am Acad Child Adolesc Psychiatry.* 2019;58(10):983–92.
4. Askelund AD, Schweizer S, Goodyer IM, van Harmelen AL. Positive memory specificity is associated with reduced vulnerability to depression. *Nat Hum Behav.* 2019;3(3):265–73.
5. Reynolds S, Orchard F, Midgley N, Kelvin R, Goodyer I, IMPACT consortium. Do sleep disturbances in depressed adolescents improve following psychological treatment for depression? *J Affect Disord.* 2020;262:205–10.
6. Khalid S, Williams CM, Reynolds SA. Is there an association between diet and depression in children and adolescents? A systematic review. *Br J Nutr.* 2016;116(12):2097–108.
7. Kandola A, Lewis G, Osborn DPJ, Stubbs B, Hayes JF. Depressive symptoms and objectively measured physical activity and sedentary behaviour throughout adolescence: a prospective cohort study. *Lancet Psychiatry.* 2020;7(3):262–71.
8. Corder K, Atkin AJ, Bamber DJ, Brage S, Dunn VJ, Ekelund U et al. Revising on the run or studying on the sofa: prospective associations between physical activity, sedentary behaviour, and exam results in British adolescents. *Int J Behav Nutr Phys Act.* 2015;12:106.

9. Corder K, van Sluijs EM, Ridgway CL, Steele RM, Prynne CJ, Stephen AM, et al. Breakfast consumption and physical activity in adolescents: daily associations and hourly patterns. *Am J Clin Nutr*. 2014;99(2):361–8.

10. Patalay P, Fitzsimons E. Correlates of mental illness and wellbeing in children: are they the same? Results from the UK Millennium Cohort Study. *J Am Acad Child Adolesc Psychiatry*. 2016;55(9):771–83.

7   BPI in Clinical Practice: Part One

In Chapters 5 and 6 we outlined the BPI framework together with clinical principles and methods. In Chapters 7 and 8 we translate these into practical BPI practice. You will have read about the concepts and techniques in prior chapters but now you get the chance to consider them through the clinical practice lens. These two chapters can serve as clinical guides and underpin the clinical manual and protocol that was used in the IMPACT study. The practice motto adopted for BPI is

Keep It Simple; Do It Well

In all respects BPI is seeking to be pragmatic, efficient and effective. This translates into keeping things simple, doing what is co-agreed with the adolescent as far as is possible but being prepared to be challenging and professionally authoritative if it means getting the best outcome for the young person.

Health and Safety

It is essential that BPI is delivered under conditions that ensure the safety of both the therapist and young person (YP). Before any clinical contact, you *must* ensure you have the following in place if you are working for a health or care provider organisation:

- a contract or agreement for working within the specific setting
- confirmation of the site-specific policies that you will need to follow (e.g. safeguarding policies on informing parents of risks identified): this is essential for discussions on confidentiality
- completion of any site-specific training (e.g. school/college-specific safeguarding training, policies on personal belongings on site, fire evacuation procedures)
- agreed plan and contact details for urgent risk advice from your service (especially how to access this when working remotely)
- site-specific named contacts for passing risk and safeguarding details on (usually the named safeguarding leads)
- contact details for parents/carers of young people aged under 18.

Core Practice Principles of BPI

Here is a recap of the key practice principles to assist the therapist to be efficient and effective in the delivery of BPI to a YP.

- Active collaboration with the YP and, where possible and clinically useful, parent(s) and other family members (e.g. siblings, grandparents, step-parents).
- The importance of establishing a trusting, collaborative relationship between the YP and the therapist.
- Mental health difficulties and associated behavioural problems should be placed within the 'lived experience' of the YP and their family.
- The developmental stage of the YP and the current phase of the family life cycle should be taken into account.
- Active encouragement to involve important others and their appropriate systems (school/college, peer group, family members) in the YP's care.
- Psychoeducation with the YP, their parents and other responsible adults to explain and help them understand current mental state, especially the differences between typical and atypical mental functions.
- Understanding mental states should be linked to advice on simple but effective ways to tackle abnormal mind and behaviour in the real world.
- Prescribing the external social world to stimulate an adaptive reorganisation of the current internal maladaptive mental state.
- Supervision is essential and is best achieved using audio clips of clinical sessions alongside BPI-specific case discussion.
- Use of measures to monitor progress session-by-session and evaluate outcomes.

Building a Collaborative Relationship in BPI

A central component of the success of any psychological therapy is generating a working collaborative alliance with the YP. There is ample evidence that such a 'therapeutic alliance' is a key factor in any psychological treatment.

For young people with mental health problems, early engagement and relationship-building is key to establishing a supportive therapeutic environment likely to be the basis for progress in treatment. When mental health problems involve depression symptoms this can be challenging because:

- Depression symptoms may cause the YP to lack motivation and struggle with social skills and prosocial behaviour.
- Often their caregivers have sought treatment for the YP so the adolescent themselves may not be help-seeking.

- Young people's expectations of adult health care professionals are likely to be based on their experiences with other adult professionals (e.g. school staff, GPs) where the adult typically has a hierarchically organised role.
- Depressed young people may well have previous experiences of loss and failure, leading them to expect therapy to fail – *remember to check their expectations at the beginning of therapy*.

Tips for clinical engagement are outlined in Table 7.1.

Table 7.1 Tips for engagement

Area	Details
Focus on the individual	Every YP is different: showing genuine curiosity about them will help you learn more and the YP will feel you really are interested in them.
Show you have kept them in mind	Keep a note of friends, family and pet names; refer back to information the YP gave in previous sessions (e.g. checking in about an exam they said was coming up).
Keep the YP central to the work	Make sure you don't get swayed too much by parents/carers: remember the YP is the most important person in your work but it can be easy to unintentionally align yourself with parents/carers when theirs are the dominant voices.
Do your homework!	Ask about the interests/hobbies of the YP, do some research about these outside of sessions, ask questions from them to learn more.
	Incorporate their interests and talents, and bring these into therapy sessions whenever you can, e.g. link healthy habits to improving performance in sports they are engaged in, recreate session worksheets with their artistic/creative input, explore favourite song lyrics relating to key BPI messages, provide further science behind healthy habits for those interested in biology.
Adapt to fit the YP	Within sessions: electronic session worksheets if handwriting is challenging, spider diagrams/cartoons of key messages, using the YP's smartphone to set reminders, saving photos of session worksheets, making use of apps that can facilitate between-session work.
	Structure/type of sessions: shorter sessions if they struggle to focus, active sessions (e.g. go for a walk, do an activity they like together), arrange timing and frequency of sessions to work around the YP's schedule and preferences.

Table 7.1 (cont.)

Area	Details
Offer your input outside of sessions and report back	Show that you are prepared to do work outside of sessions, just as you expect the YP to do between-session activities, e.g. send a letter to school/college confirming appointments to reduce the stress of explaining this to school staff, research pastoral support options in the college they are due to start at.
Be creative!!	Activation is a central component in BPI, so as long as you are helping the YP activate themselves and make positive changes in their behaviour, you can do this in many different ways.

Creating a Culture That Can Be Helpful

We have emphasised the importance of a collaborative working alliance for clinical effectiveness. The purpose is to create a clinical culture that can be helpful to the YP. Without this it is likely that effective implementation will be reduced. Table 7.2 shows key components that we consider create a helpful therapeutic alliance.

Table 7.2 Principles of creating a collaborative alliance with the young person

Principles to encourage/foster	Attitudes to counter/challenge
Balanced optimism: communicating a belief that things can get better for the YP although it may be gradual and at times challenging	Pessimism and hopelessness
Educating: understanding mental states and their functions	Illness beliefs and behaviours
Activation: encouraging a position of action and solution for the YP and family	Helplessness and inertia
Problem-solving: identifying problems and working together to consider possible solutions and plan solution attempts	Helplessness and passivity
Listening and support: hearing the YP's lived experience, not judging, providing positive reinforcement for all attempts to improve their situation	Telling them what to do, not listening to the YP's voice

BPI Structure

Brief psychosocial intervention has been designed to be flexible so the stages and clinical tools can be selected as appropriate for the actual lived process, rather than sessions having to take place in a specific order. The overarching aim is to help the YP take control of their mental health and behaviour and work on what is most important to them. For the therapist the flexibility allows them to select from the toolbox the techniques that fit the YP best. The BPI therapist should feel confident in revisiting areas of uncertainty or misunderstanding if these arise and ensuring that the objectives of the therapy have the best chance of being achieved. Indeed, clinical effectiveness is likely best achieved by the therapist checking and reinforcing success and, where required, revisiting areas that need further improvement to effect the best habilitation for the YP. There are some mandatory topics that we have observed from practice and research which we consider enhance the likelihood of BPI being effective. These are:

- getting to know you (some initial information-gathering is essential but this can be supplemented later on if the YP takes some time to feel comfortable sharing information with you)
- keeping you safe (risk assessment and management)
- understanding mental states as a key component of psychoeducation
- prosocial and personal activity: external social and personal performance change that leads to a normalising internal mental state
- review and ending.

These five mandatory interviewing procedures can be easily carried out within the three practice steps of 'getting to know you', 'taking active steps' and 'bringing it all together'. The hypothesised relationships between practice and theory principles are shown in Figure 7.1.

These represent areas of theoretical knowledge, content and practical strategy that the BPI therapist will select tools and techniques from. Note that both theoretically and in practice therapists must be prepared to retrace some steps where there is an apparent lack of clarity, understanding or progress. Habilitative strategies are likely necessary to ensure that there has been sufficient learning by the adolescent to reduce symptoms and improve their personal functions and overall well-being.

The ten elements are found distributed under each of the practice headings as shown in Figure 7.2.

As we have noted, these elements are not to be implemented in any particular sequence or order as this is not a rigid delivery protocol but a mental and behavioural toolbox which the therapist will use according to each individual case need. The objective, therefore, is to consider BPI as a clinical intervention

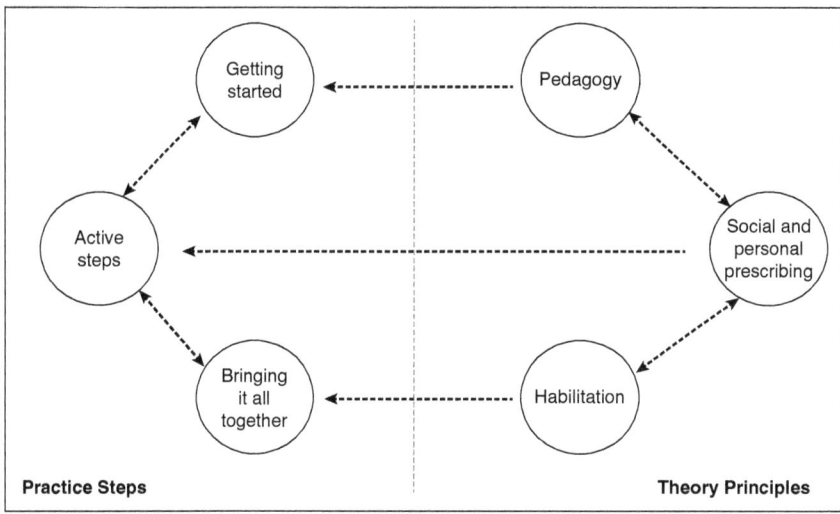

Figure 7.1 Practice framework and theory principles

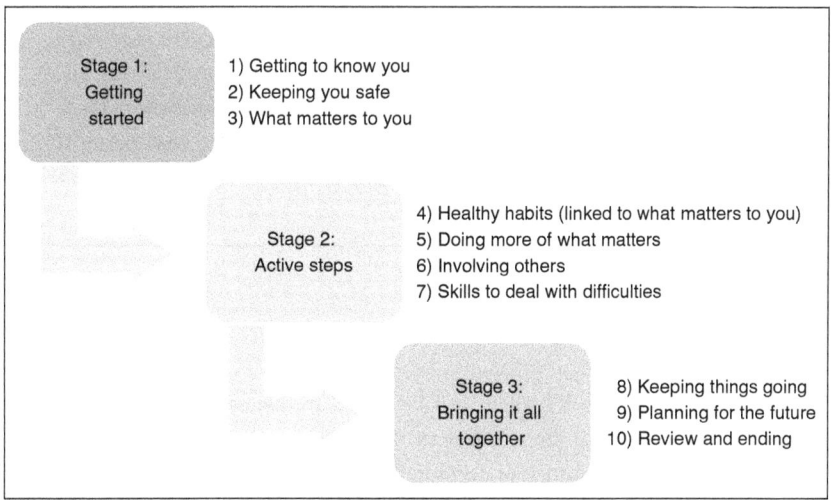

Figure 7.2 Practice domains and tools

whose component parts can be used flexibly and collaboratively, with the needs of the YP being paramount. Using a collaborative working alliance will be the process that in part determines the pace and clinical change and will signal to the BPI therapist which of the clinical tools in the framework will be selected for the intervention at any one time over the course of therapy. Evaluating the pace and change with the YP will be based on the collaborative working alliance between therapist and YP.

Clinical Example

Dan and the therapist had determined that social isolation was not good for his mental health despite Dan reporting that his mental state appeared to suggest that his friends did not want him around currently because he was not a 'good' person to be with. At the previous session Dan had admitted that he was struggling to meet with others outside of school hours despite saying he would try as agreed. The therapist decided to revisit the psychoeducational element that had formed the basis of the social prescribing (pedagogic review). *It was clear that Dan had not remembered enough about understanding mental states and how an unwell mind may not be giving good advice. The therapist and Dan went over the importance of understanding his current mental state and learning and embedding that an unwell mind can give bad advice, recalling this new understanding for the purpose of prosocial activity* (habilitation). *The activity plan* (social prescribing) *was also reviewed collaboratively but it was agreed to try again with the current activity of friendship re-engagement, with Dan remembering to recall his understanding of current mental state to reduce social withdrawing mood, thoughts and behaviours, thereby aiding social activity. The therapist also reminded Dan that it requires behavioural effort to engage with friends; passivity will not work.*

Confidentiality

In getting to know the YP, there is a key need to discuss the rules governing confidentiality and the circumstances that may result in the need to break these. Given the importance of confidentiality, this discussion should occur at the very start of the first meeting with the YP (and/or parent or carer). It may be helpful to repeat this at the start of the next few sessions and to remind the YP of this discussion if you need to break confidentiality. Table 7.3 outlines a script as a guide for discussing confidentiality. Figure 7.3 highlights when it is you might need to consider breaking confidentiality, only after careful discussion in liaison with a senior colleague. Table 7.4 shows a pathway of action should a risk be identified and Figure 7.4 summarises the risk foci that may be revealed in a conversational treatment.

Table 7.3 Guide for discussing confidentiality

Example confidentiality (and limits) script

'Before we start, I'd like to tell you what kind of things we can discuss and keep confidential – that means private. What we talk about together is confidential. Most of the time I'm not going to tell your parents, friends, teachers or other people you know what you've told me if you don't want me to … but there are times we do need to share information and we'll talk about that.

'We share information in our team to make sure we're giving you the best care possible, but we do this in a way that means it is still kept private from other people.

'It's often also helpful to share a lot of what we talk about together with important people in your life so they can support you in the most helpful way, but there might be things you want to keep between us which, for most of the time, is fine.

'But there are times when I would need to tell someone else what you've told me, even if you don't want me to. If I was worried about your safety, or the safety of someone else, I would have to share the information to help keep you or the other person safe. Who I share the information with depends on the exact situation, but I might have to share this with your parents, your GP or other adults.

'I would always talk to you before doing this so that we could come up with a plan together, like me being with you while you share the information, or me sharing the information for you. Does this sound ok? Do you have any questions?'

Identifying a risk to the YP sets in motion a clinical procedure with the YP that we have outlined in a sequential step process shown in Table 7.4.

Occasionally, a YP may not consent to sharing a risk situation with important others such as parents. The therapist must then consider whether breaking confidentiality is justified in the best interests of the YP. When such a decision may have to be taken is shown in Figure 7.3.

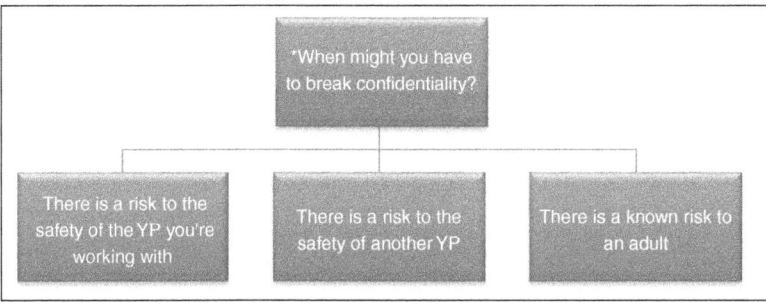

Figure 7.3 When might you have to break confidentiality?

Table 7.4 Process to follow if risk is identified

Reminder of confidentiality & limits	• Recap what was previously said about confidentiality and limits to this. • Check if any adults already aware of risk (explain you will need to speak to them anyway, can't assume they know even if YP says so).
Explore positives of sharing with YP's consent	Explain that by sharing this information with adults involved in their care you feel it will help keep them/other person if risk relates to someone else safe, so you would like to do so. Highlight positives of risk sharing: - Others understanding YP's difficulties more fully. - Not having to keep these difficulties to themselves and dealing with them alone. - Others being able to help keep them safe (e.g. providing extra support when needed, reducing chance of impulsive acts by removing access to means).
Explore YP's view of potential negatives of risk sharing	Explore YP's view of potential negatives of risk sharing, e.g: - Parents/carers 'over-reacting': explain your training and ability to share information in a normalising, validating way. - Extra stress/burden on parent/carer: explain this is part of being a parent and feedback indicates they would much rather know. - *Any signs indicating that sharing risk information will increase risk itself.*
If YP consents to risk information sharing	• Agree their preferred way of sharing risk, exactly what information to be shared, with whom and when. • Document this discussion and sharing of risk clearly in clinical notes.
If YP does not consent to risk information sharing	• Explain you have a duty of care to act in their best interests. • State you will need to speak to a supervisor to discuss what needs to happen next. • Seek immediate support from a senior colleague or supervisor, if necessary as a break during the session. • If you are concerned about a YP's ability to keep themselves safe in the *immediate* future, do not leave them alone or allow them to leave without gaining advice from a senior colleague/supervisor. • Document the discussion with YP, input from senior colleague/supervisor and agreed actions clearly in clinical notes.

The key issue that needs to be considered is the best interests of the YP: weight of risk vs potential negative outcomes of breaking confidentiality in the absence of informed consent to do so. You will need to follow service and site-specific policies on this, which may vary between organisations such as hospital settings, community health clinics and schools.

Assessing and Managing Risks for Suicidality and Self-Harming Behaviours

Once suicidality and/or self-harm risk (SSHR) has been identified there must be a clear clinical management plan. BPI offers a set of general principles for therapists to follow:

- SSHR assessment and management take priority over any other content.
- If you have any concerns about how to manage SSHR arising in session, seek supervision. (It is ok to do this during the session if you are not confident the YP should be allowed to go home.)
- When seeing a YP with their parent/carer, always allow time for exploration of SSHR alone with the YP.
- Performing repeated SSHR assessments alone may identify the 'risk' but not change it: therapists should focus on understanding the dangers and making progress on actions to modify risk once it has been clearly confirmed.

Asking explicitly about current and past suicidal thoughts and self-harming acts is a key aspect of revealing and then discussing current SSHR. Identifying and assessing the impact of hazardous behaviours on the YP is a first step to providing an explanatory framework for reducing such risks. BPI therapists should establish: *why* is the YP doing it and what purpose does it serve? Is there a more helpful (and less harmful) way of getting this need met? Some important features of SSHR evaluation are as follows:

- Severity of depression and other mental illnesses can be an indicator of risk but additional factors can increase this (e.g. interpersonal difficulties, thoughts of hopelessness).
- It is important to differentiate between self-harm aimed at providing some kind of relief/communication/change (non-suicidal) and self-harm aimed at ending life or endangering life (suicidal).
  - It is critical to explore the aim and intent of any risky actions, regardless of the level of lethality.

- The more detached and isolated, hopeless and entrapped the YP appears, the greater the risk is likely to be.
  ○ External difficulties may be contributors: for example, distressing family circumstances, personal educational failures at school or negative peer group interactions may be increasing suicidal thoughts and/or self-harming behaviours. In these cases, there is a need to evaluate and directly address the adverse environmental circumstances. A clinical relationship that may be present between internal risky thoughts and external difficulties is shown in Figure 7.4, which also depicts the additive effects of risks in mental state and the environment that may increase the transition from suicidal thoughts to acts.

Managing Self-Harm and Suicidality

- Provide concrete advice to the YP and family on managing risk (e.g. removing means of harm, increasing supervision, identifying triggers and warning signs).
- Share information to help others keep the YP safe.
- Provide a trusting relationship and a place to be understood.
- Look for solutions to crises/problems that lead to SSHR.

Factors Indicating Potential Increased Suicidality in Young People Who Also Self-Harm

- Older teenage male
- Violent self-harm method
- Multiple episodes of self-harm

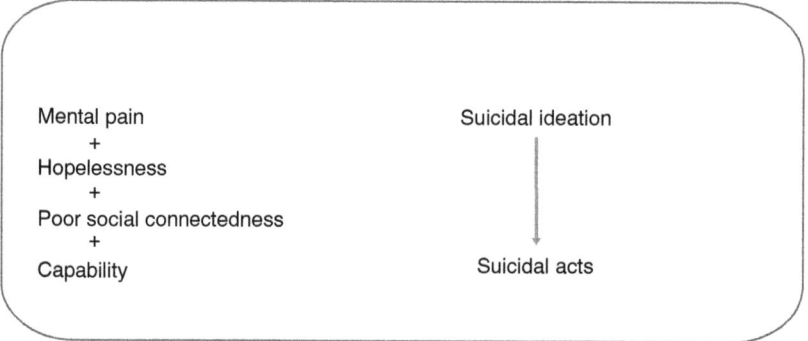

Figure 7.4 Potential additive effects of mental components on risk for suicide

- Apathy (lack of interest, enthusiasm, or concern)
- Hopelessness
- Insomnia
- Substance misuse
- Previous psychiatric hospital admission
- Behaviour disorder

Creating a Collaborative Safety Plan

We recommend completing a safety plan collaboratively with the YP as part of the therapeutic activity. This should set out principles of action the YP can take when they feel overwhelmed by current events and experience anger, irritability or distress. A safety plan should be in place for all in therapy even if the YP does not have current experience of suicidal ideation or urges to self-harm. In addition to the safety plan, therapists should take advantage of the risk management guidelines shown in Table 7.4, selecting the components that fit the individual YP they are working with at the time. We suggest a set of practical interventions for BPI safety planning, which is detailed in Table 7.5.

Liaison with Other Services

The rules of consent and confidentiality apply to all information-sharing but it's helpful for therapists to emphasise the benefits of joining up support. There are likely to be important points of interaction with other important persons and organisations as therapy proceeds. Indeed, as BPI uses external strategies in the YP's environment to evoke internal change in the current mental state, connecting with others is to be expected.

Parent/Carer and Other Adult Involvement

A key role of the therapist in BPI is to help the YP gain support from important adults in their life, and for them to understand how they can best help. This includes:

- inviting parents/carers into some part of BPI sessions (e.g. the last ten minutes), providing BPI resources, arranging phone calls if they are unable to attend sessions

Table 7.5 SSHR management guidelines

Risk management action	Why this is important
Advise parents/carers to remove access to means of harm.	Removing access to means of harm is a simple way to reduce young people acting on impulse. Medication especially is often left around the home (parents are usually unaware of how lethal these can be, e.g. paracetamol).
Focus on what the YP feels would be helpful: this sometimes means parents agreeing to leave them alone when they are upset (e.g. not going into their bedroom when their child is upset but texting their child to check if they are ok).	To help the YP feel heard by the therapist and their family; to agree on a balance of appropriate supervision without intrusive behaviour.
Explore the use of code words or numbers to facilitate risk communication between young people and parents, e.g. 0–10 rating scale for mood check-in, agreement of at what number parents need to intervene (e.g. 'anything below a 4 needs mum to help me keep myself safe').	There may be conflict or a lack of communication in families, which makes sharing risk difficult, and these are hard conversations for anyone to have. Giving a shorthand reduces some of the barriers and agreeing with a therapist helps the YP feel their parent/carer will listen to them.
Try to encourage the YP to reach out to important adults rather than friends and ensure these adults have a copy of their safety plan.	Other young people may struggle to cope with this emotional burden and may be experiencing difficulties themselves.
Bring any cases where risk has been identified to supervision.	To ensure you as a therapist have support in managing this and to explore whether any other input is needed for the YP.
Follow up risk management strategies with YP and family.	To check these have been implemented and are working; to problem-solve any barriers; this information helps evaluate the level of risk.

- providing important adults with psychoeducation about mental states and psychopathology, such as depression in young people, and the particular difficulties their adolescent faces
- supporting the YP to make use of the network of adults around them to facilitate their recovery
- problem-solving any barriers adults may present to the YP making progress in BPI
- negotiating information-sharing between the YP and adults, and therapist risk information.

Finally, if you are having any contact with adults when the YP is not present, always aim to inform the YP about this so they do not feel you are 'going behind their back'.

Liaising with important others and services is a clinical and an operational skill. Like many clinical skills, it improves with experience but even practitioners with much experience face challenges in liaison. Table 7.6 provides a guide to the common challenges any therapist can face. Figure 7.5 shows the other services that a YP may be exposed to and that a BPI therapist may need to engage with to ensure clinical effectiveness.

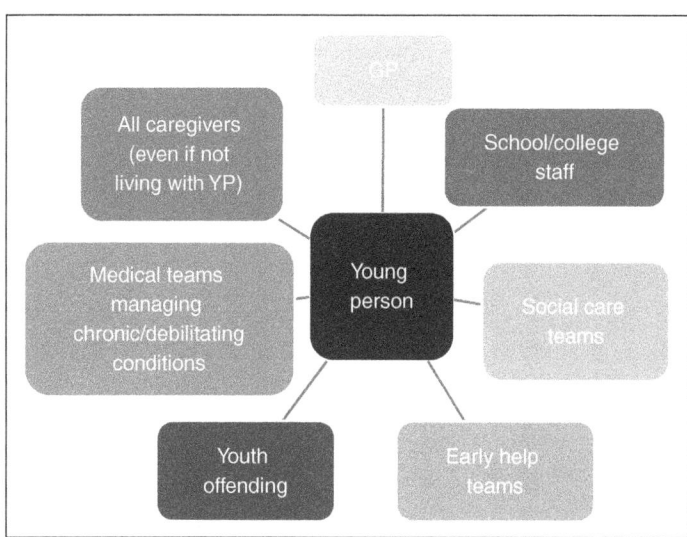

Figure 7.5   Key liaison domains

Table 7.6 shows the five challenges to be aware of when involving others and suggests potential solutions.

Table 7.6 Challenges of involving others and potential solutions

Challenge of involving others	Potential solution
The YP does not want parents/carers involved.	Discuss the possible ways to involve parents/carers without sharing personal details (e.g. providing them with handouts, having general conversations about BPI content without specifics relating to the YP); agree on what can/can't be shared; explore reasons behind this and problem-solve if there are any barriers that can be easily overcome; find out if there are other important adults that could be involved instead of parents/carers (e.g. aunt, grandfather, older adult sibling, step-parent, school pastoral lead, college tutor). Review involvement of others regularly as YP's initial reluctance could reduce through therapy.
Parents/carers do not appear motivated to be involved.	Directly request input from parents/carers in BPI; emphasise this is a central part of treatment; discuss ways to make this as feasible as possible (e.g. if childcare/work commitments make coming to sessions difficult, arrange a phone call or email updates).
Significant conflict between the YP and adults who may be central to supporting their recovery.	Use BPI content of contracts and problem-solving to explore this with the YP and adult(s); emphasise that improving relationships is central to the YP's recovery. Be mindful that in cases of serious, escalating conflict there may be safeguarding issues – bring any concerns to supervision.
The parent/carer has their own mental health problem, which makes it hard for them to support the YP in making progress.	Mental illnesses such as depression are often familial. It is therefore important to explore with parents/carers their own mental health and those of grandparents both now and in the past. For parents with current mental health problems, emphasise the importance of seeking help for themselves and support them to do so. This may be aiding consultations for them with primary care or mental health services. Encourage parents/carers to make use of the BPI principles as a family (e.g. healthy eating, doing more of what matters, etc.).
It is difficult to get the parent/carer to complete planned actions between sessions.	Consider ways you can make this easier for parents/carers: for example, increase communication, emphasising their value and importance in therapy; get the YP to check in on potential actions for parents/carers before agreeing on them; explore who else might be able to complete actions if parents/carers cannot (e.g. the therapist making direct contact with school staff to discuss their support, with parent/carer permission).

8   BPI in Clinical Practice: Part Two

The Importance of Psychoeducation

We want to emphasise the importance of psychoeducation (PE) as an active intervention in clinical BPI practice. As noted already, PE was originally considered as a passive aid to medical treatments rather than an active therapeutic agent. For example, it is highly likely that PE enhances adherence and collaborative working in any intervention through explaining the implications of treatment to the patient. This is undoubtedly a useful mediating process but in BPI practice we want the therapist to utilise PE from the perspective that it acts as a therapeutic change element of treatment. For BPI practice, PE is the conversational delivery vehicle for information about how to understand mental states, engage in adaptive activities and habilitate and use new understandings and strategies to promote well-being and resilience in the face of future adversities. Whilst the focus is directly on the adolescent, such PE can also be delivered to important others such as family, carers and teachers, with the consent of the YP.

Clinical Example

Getting to Know You: Initiating a Working Collaboration with a Worried Young Adolescent

Thirteen-year-old Amy arrived at the clinic with her mother. On entering the clinical office, she sat on the same chair as mum and would not look directly at the therapist. The therapist began by introducing herself and what she was planning to do. The first interview questions would be to mum as Amy was a little uncertain about the surroundings (didactic clear communication of focus for information-gathering). *She asked Amy if this was ok with her; Amy moved closer to mum and nodded briefly but did not look up. The therapist embarked on 15 minutes of information-gathering in a systematic and structured manner regarding mum's understanding of Amy's presenting problems, the well-being of family members in the household and her medical history. Amy was regularly asked (every five minutes) if mum was getting things right and she nodded*

---

in assent each time. The therapist made no attempt to engage Amy further on each occasion; indeed, she thanked Amy for confirming the history and returned to mum with no attempt to draw Amy out of herself.

After the information-gathering Amy volunteered without being asked that the family had a dog and a cat who lived at home as these had not been recorded. The therapist asked Amy directly (didactic questioning) *if the animals were well and if there were any other family members who had been left out. Amy looked up directly at the therapist and said no. The therapist asked the name of the dog and the cat and if Amy had any photographs on her phone. Amy gave the name of the dog (George) and cat (Cindy) and showed a photo of George. The therapist thanked Amy and said if it was ok with her, it was time to talk about what was going on in her mind. The therapist said it would be great if Amy would answer some questions directly* (didactic refocus on the adolescent) *but mum could chip in and help too. Amy hesitated but said 'ok'. The therapist moved the didactic information-gathering focus to Amy and said that together they should make sure mum did not chip in unless Amy wanted her help.*

This 'getting to know you' vignette illustrates the important clinical beginning for using PE to help the YP understand current mental state and how mental illnesses may disrupt efficient functioning in the mind and disrupt both personal and social behaviour. Indeed, a large part of BPI throughout the intervention is helping the YP and their family to understand the nature of mental illnesses such as depression. Part of PE is to be clear that the YP can improve their understanding of mental states and make adaptive behavioural changes by overcoming the barrier of the mental illness. Psychoeducation must be clear that BPI is effortful and is likely to involve going to the 'mental gym' to return the mind to a state of well-being.

Clinical Example

Understanding Mental States

Abdullah, aged 15 years, came to the clinic with his parents. Abdullah had willingly engaged with the therapist, declaring he did not like the 'state he was in' and wanted to get back to the way he was before 'all this happened'. The therapist and he had agreed that in the next meeting they would explore Abdullah's current mental state and see what might be learned from doing this. At the second meeting Abdullah was asked to describe his current mood, thoughts, feelings and sensations, with the BPI therapist interjecting to improve clarity and coherence. Abdullah said that he felt 'numb and empty' rather than depressed, sad or irritable. He said it was all the time and had crept up on him slowly and was noticed by friends, but he did not want to talk to them about his feelings. He then said he was having trouble getting off to sleep and was beginning to think he was a 'weirdo' because he could not concentrate and 'kept wandering off in his head to nowhere in particular'. He did not understand what was going on – the more time he spent thinking about it, the less sense it made. He could not figure out what to do and kind of felt 'done in' by it all.

The BPI therapist began the session by asking Abdullah if he had wondered about where all these 'mind' features he had described might come from. He thought about this and said he knew they were part of his mind and not 'aliens' but how they came to be with him all the time he did not know. Abdullah thought a bit more about this and then said that these mental things occurring all together and sticking around in his head was the weird bit. Abdullah continued: 'Yeah, I can get, like, down sometimes and I can have, like, negative thoughts, and everyone has bad sleep sometimes, but having all these things, like, together is really weird.'

The therapist said, 'Your mind seems all cluttered up – you cannot think straight!' Abdullah replied, saying, 'Yeah, that's right, I cannot think straight – stuff keeps going round and round and won't go away and I cannot concentrate on normal stuff, which makes me angry.' The therapist said, 'So what you want, then, is to straighten out your mind and get it moving again?' Abdullah: 'Yeah, I guess so. I never thought about my mind before. I guess it's just like, yeah, me, isn't it?' The therapist said,: 'Mental states getting stuck like yours is part of the mental illness, so this is not your fault. That's really important to understand.' Abdullah: 'Oh, so, like, being like this is, like, part of the illness and not me then? Ok, so what do I do about that then?' The therapist replied, 'First, we need to have you remember that your mind is not always on your side. When it is unwell you are less likely to think straight – your moods, thoughts and feelings/sensations tend to clutter up your mental space, as you now appreciate.' The therapist checked with Abdullah to ensure he had understood.

Psychoeducation (PE) is not focused on the YP's mental state alone. It is also about getting important others to understand the YP's mental state and the value of a personal sense of achievement and prosocial behaviours in aiding mental recovery. The clinical vignette above was a first step in engaging in a mental state conversation with Abdullah's parents and older brother, with his full consent. Abdullah stayed for this PE conversation on understanding mental states. The therapist ensured that all family members had grasped as much as possible from this conversation. The therapist also made it clear that they could have further family sessions if needed to clarify and check what had been learned about the mind when well and ill (habilitation). Involving parents and enabling them to understand mental states and support their adolescent as they work to regain well-being is a critical element in PE. In Table 8.1 we outline PE principles to aid understanding of mental states, the YP's environment and how important others can aid recovery.

Table 8.1 Psychoeducation can enhance protective factors and build resilience

If parent(s) are supportive and willing to help	Emphasise how important this can be, e.g. encouraging social behaviours, speaking to school, co-planning healthy habits such as regular sleep patterns and doing family activities together.
If the YP has retained interest in an activity/hobby	Highlight the therapeutic effect of engaging in an activity that matters to the adolescent. Reflect and reinforce that a positive impact on well-being can accrue from a specific activity/hobby that is rewarding.
If the YP has positive friendships	Discuss the importance of social connection despite the barrier of depression and other mental symptoms. Encourage engagement with social groups and expanding types/frequency of social activities.
If the YP has access to facilitating resources	Discuss the benefits of these resources (e.g. owns a bike, family friend is a tennis coach, sibling is studying catering, lives close to amenities) and how to make the most of them.
If the YP has existing strategies for well-being	Explore what has helped or could help that's already in their wellbeing toolkit. Discuss if these can be built on in simple ways (e.g. doing them more frequently, scheduling them, in creating a routine).

Clinical Example

Taking Actions for Well-Being: Social Prescribing

Nina was angry, argumentative and often sullen. Her parents felt she had lost interest in them; they felt hurt, rejected and angry and Nina was 'online all the time or hanging out with her new mates', whom her parents hardly knew. Self-harm seemed to be part of the 'culture' of these new friends: her parents were concerned. They felt she was 16 now and making her own way, but some of the style, culture and behaviour came as a bit of shock.

Nina was dismissive of the meeting, feeling it was other people who had made her come. The therapist quickly realised Nina was at risk of disengaging and decided it was especially important to spend time getting to know Nina: the Nina now and the Nina of one, two and three years ago. This timeline work helped to formulate Nina's recent behaviour. There was evidence of a step-change coinciding with the onset of a clinical depression followed by episodes of self-harm. Nina volunteered that she used to like shooting a basketball and was once a keen artist, loving drawing and making things. She no longer did this and she said she had drifted away from the friends she used to have.

Nina's maternal grandmother had died a couple of years back and mum had taken this loss badly. Already stressed and overworked, mum and Nina started squabbling and arguing about everyday things: little hassles became big problems and Nina retreated from family functions and stopped communicating with her mum and dad.

The therapist suggested to Nina that she experiment with messing about on the basketball court again: a long-time hobby she had given up a year previously. She also suggested mum and Nina find a few minutes to do something together in 'parallel': not necessarily 'to talk' but to 'do something together, anything, even washing-up or a walk with the dog', just to be with each other and share the activity, like they used to. Nina seemed curious and some lightening of her mood and expression was noted by the therapist as they toyed with these ideas. Collaboratively they spent time getting the right type of activity and amount of time to share with mum.

In the following session Nina reported that she had bumped into an old mate and spontaneously ended up messing about on the basketball court. Nina said, 'It felt good, it reminded me how much fun it used to be' and 'I felt a bit different'.

Mum said Nina and she had found time to do something they had both forgotten about, life drawing, and they hadn't squabbled whilst engaging with this together – in fact they had a chuckle about each other's sketches and agreed to do it again next week.

Nina's mood was brightening; she was still low and still self-harming but this had decreased in frequency.

Nina's therapist was encouraged that her formulation was on the right track and the social prescribing action plan was already bearing fruit. She had a feeling, indeed she hypothesised in her formulation, that on this improvement trajectory Nina would gradually stop self-harming and shift friendship groups.

Working Out Where to Focus the Social Prescribing Activity Work

Activity is 'prescribed', collaboratively, in BPI at every opportunity, including during but also following 'getting to know you', and imparting through PE an understanding of mental states.

As we have emphasised, in BPI the therapist develops the intervention plan collaboratively with the YP and, where possible, with family support. Consideration of where (and when) to intervene should be based on:

(i)   The likely benefit arising from:
   - decreasing the exposure to a risk factor (e.g. drinking alcohol, arguments with parents)
   - increasing resilience (e.g. building up a support network amongst family and friends and on occasion other important adults including teachers)
   - amplifying protective factors (e.g. increasing physical activity, enhancing personal hobbies and interests)
   - paying particular attention to the severity of and hazards associated with the disorder by reducing suicidality or self-harm ideation and substance misuse

- attention to addressing risk to others, such as the presence of antisocial behaviours.
(ii) The likelihood of the proposed intervention/s achieving this benefit. This means choosing the tools and techniques most likely to be clinically effective.
(iii) The likelihood of those involved engaging in the proposed intervention.
    - There should be a collaborative working relationship with the YP and the family.
    - There should be a view regarding prognosis and what outcomes might be hoped for.
    - There should be a plan for when to review and how to measure progress and a clear collaborative understanding of how and when therapy will end.

All of this is part of formulation and should ideally be recorded briefly in the case file and working notes. This will help you as a therapist to work through your thoughts and crystallise your next steps. It will also support service quality assurance and provide an auditable trail of clinical decision-making. That will help you as a therapist to learn from every case that you treat and for the service to learn more broadly. Most importantly it will help you to remember and formulate understanding and action to the benefit of your patient.

Supporting Young People to Record Their Activity

Most young people with mental health problems such as depression will struggle to engage in between-session ('homework') activities due to the nature of their mental disorder. It is important that the therapist recognises this and works collaboratively to aim for realistic and achievable between-session tasks. It is *essential* that these tasks are arrived at collaboratively and comprehensively explained in session. An example of what is being agreed on as a task should be gone through and rehearsed so that there is a clear understanding of what is expected and what the goal is that the YP has agreed to try to achieve. Tips for activity monitoring are given in Table 8.2.

Working with What Matters to the Young Person

Establishing what matters and developing a clear understanding of these is a way into many aspects of healthy habits and can help increase motivation for effortful activity. As these are identified by the YP themselves, this can lead to improved mental health and more positive mental health supporting behaviours: for example, 'I want to eat healthily', 'Getting a good night's sleep

Table 8.2 Key tips for explaining activity monitoring

Allocate sufficient time in session to explain the rationale and go through an example fully.	Adapt activity monitoring to the YP (personalise frequency, duration, detail and ratings as well as method of recording).
Explain the key role of this task = a way of getting to know the YP better, learn more about them.	Encourage any effort and set expectations low, use parental support/facilitation of task if the YP finds this acceptable.
Be aware this process can be confronting for some young people (having their mental health problems clearly revealed). Discuss how to use new understanding as a step towards positive change.	Think about what the YP might want to record, e.g. activities, meals, sleep, exercise.
Link back to key rationale in BPI: small changes can make a big difference so you need the detail to find where these small changes could happen.	Check understanding and level of engagement before setting homework task.

is important to me'. Some things that matter may indicate areas of tension between current behaviour and how the YP says they want to live (e.g. current substance use conflicts with 'Looking after myself') so they can be a way into discussing unhelpful behaviours. It is important to recognise that what matters most to a YP may not be the same as a therapist's view or their parent's/carer's, sibling's and peer's views; however, activities that matter to the YP should be encouraged in all instances, except where there are direct negative consequences or they are known to be harmful (e.g. drug-taking, going directly against reasonable family rules). Any concern over such issues should be taken to supervision.

Activities that go beyond healthy habits per se are likely to be prosocial and external so that the YP is enhancing or reconnecting with their peer network or re-engaging with their family. These should of course be encouraged. Additionally, however, it is important to examine and consider the need to work collaboratively on personal hobbies, interests and pastimes. These personal interests and potential achievement domains can also include educational and technical skills goals.

Working on Healthy Habits

Why Is Sleep Important?

Sleep difficulties were the most frequently reported symptom amongst depressed adolescents in the IMPACT study and are common in adolescents with mood-related mental health problems regardless of diagnosis [1–3]. Sleep difficulties during adolescence are also associated with mental health difficulties during young adulthood. Psychological treatment of the depression will reduce sleep difficulties in many cases so monitoring and attending to sleep hygiene is part of BPI and is therefore an important clinical strategy.

Clinical Example

Marcus, aged 16 years, came for his third session of BPI and reported that he was beginning to get the idea about his mental state not being on his side, as it were, when he was mentally unwell. He said it was hard to appreciate but he was getting there. He and the therapist began to talk about doing things that were good for Marcus. These included a discussion about healthy habits where Marcus said that he still had trouble with sleeping. This was at much the same level of difficulty as when BPI started. Collaboratively, the therapist and Marcus put together his current sleep patterns. This analysis first showed there really was not any consistency in bedtime routines. Further, there was no predictable bedroom environment and what was there was clearly wakeful: this included a games console, mobile phone and tablet. Marcus joked that, although he might go to bed at 11, his social media never slept. The therapist also established that the room had curtains that let in plenty of light and that the bedroom door was poorly fitting and often open to the hallway and house noise. The BPI tool for the therapist here is 'environmental prescribing'; a list of agreed themes was:

- *Develop a sleep hygiene pattern that is consistent in routine.*
- *Make sure the bedroom is quiet, dark, relaxing and at a comfortable temperature.*
- *Remove from the bedroom or at a minimum immobilise electronic devices such as TVs, computers and smartphones.*
- *Avoid large meals, caffeine and alcohol before bedtime.*

These were reviewed in the subsequent session and Marcus was helped to problem-solve to keep things moving forwards as indeed his sleep patterns began to regularise and improve.

Why Is Nutrition Important?

The association between depression and eating is predominantly one of the mental illness influencing a reduction in overall eating and a lowering of nutritional elements in the diet.

Clinical Example

Gina, 15 years old, had been seeing the BPI therapist for six weeks, having received three sessions at fortnightly intervals. She had been referred for depressed mood and loss of energy associated with a change in habit, including a loss of interest in eating. She was highly motivated to get better, had enjoyed learning about her mind and was good at understanding her mental state. She had rejoined her friends and was getting on better with her schoolwork but was struggling with eating. The therapist suggested they spend the first part of this session examining both her eating patterns and the nutritional elements of her diet. Gina noted that she had lost her appetite and therefore, from the eating habit perspective, she was forgetting to eat in the manner she usually did. She said she was not especially interested in food and saw it more as 'fuel for life' than an interesting thing to do. Because of this, she admitted, she was simply eating 'on the go', grabbing whatever was available and paying no attention to what she was eating. Gina did say that this 'grab and go' eating style was very likely to be less good for her than regular meals at breakfast, lunch and dinner. Further discussion revealed this was a pattern and style that was not present prior to her mental illness.

Although she could not imagine herself becoming a 'foodie', she agreed with the therapist that getting back to eating how she had before would be better than what was happening right now. This eating analysis led to Gina planning to eat meals rather than snacking randomly and to include foods she liked without having to 'experiment' at this time.

Gina agreed to keep a written record of the times she took her meals in relation to waking and going to bed. Gina also noted what she ate and agreed this was currently a priority for her now that she was getting back into the life that she had before becoming clinically depressed.

The therapist wanted Gina to also note her mental state in relation to eating time or food content, which she agreed to do. Gina's mum was invited into the session to be made aware of the activity plan and to provide any comments and thoughts. Mum agreed, with Gina's permission, to act as an additional recorder of mealtimes and food content in relation to waking and bedtimes. They agreed to go shopping together to get a set of foods that Gina was willing to eat. This reconnecting of mum and Gina was an added benefit to Gina's therapeutic progress in BPI, and entirely in keeping with the BPI prosocial, recovery-oriented stance.

Two weeks later at her fourth session, she reported that it had been hard to return to mealtimes rather than snacks and her mother's support had been very important. Gina also said her mum had helped her regarding what to buy to eat. Gina said, though, that if her mental state had not already been on the mend she doubted if she would have been able to change her eating habits. She said she 'learned a lot' about eating and well-being over the last few weeks, and her and mum's relationship was also getting back to 'how it used to be'.

Here are some guidance points when assessing eating, diet and nutrition:

- There is a very wide range of diets and knowledge about nutrition in young people. So it is important not to assume they know the basics of what a healthy vs unhealthy diet is.
- Exploring diet and nutrition can help flag up any other difficulties around eating (e.g. physical health concerns, cognitions indicating a desire for thinness that require more specialist assessment) as well as social adversity (e.g. parental neglect or poverty as barriers to adequate nutrition).
- Be careful not to prescribe changes in nutrition without expert knowledge. The evidence for direct causal links between poor diet and the onset of mental illness in adolescents is not robust.
- Key issues are to avoid over- or under-eating and support a balanced nutritional health approach to available foods.

Why Are Drugs and Alcohol Important?

The use of illicit drugs, smoking and alcohol amongst adolescents is difficult to quantify but perhaps 25% to 35% of adolescents in developed countries are users, with 10% to 20% being regular and frequent users and compromising their well-being as a result [4, 5]. Illicit drug use is associated with many negative health, social and economic consequences and is a significant contributor to three of the leading causes of death among young persons (aged 10 to 24 years): unintentional injuries, including motor vehicle crashes, suicide and homicide.

This makes assessing drug, smoking and alcohol use an important part of the 'getting to know you' phase of BPI. In adolescents with mental health problems, monitoring the use of these substances during treatment is also important. There are no reliable predictors of substance use in depressed adolescents currently undergoing treatment so the therapist must maintain an open evaluation stance towards these behaviours as treatment progresses. We cannot assume that improvements in mental health will mean concurrent reductions in any substance use.

Here are the principles of assessment and intervention for adolescent patients with mental health problems where substance use is of concern:

- There are significant associations between depression and smoking, alcohol and substance misuse [6].
- Many services have NHS Trust-specific policies on offering smoking cessation and other substance advice programmes; often these are not offered to young people due to an assumption that they are not required or a reluctance to ask difficult questions.
- Substance use in adolescence is associated with a range of other risk factors. For example, it may indicate family/peer substance use, adverse early life events or low parental involvement.
- Substance misuse also increases the chances of risky behaviour, including suicidal ideation and completed suicide.
- A young person who is using drugs or alcohol may struggle to engage in psychological therapy and require more specialised input to deal with addiction and dependency issues.
- Often young people may use drugs or alcohol as an unhelpful coping strategy, so recognising this and linking it to making choices and healthy habits can identify more helpful strategies.

Why Is Digital/Online Life Important?

There is considerable expansion and worldwide use of social media by young people and a small but significant association between frequent use and risk to mental health [7]. Amongst adolescents, there are views that suggest that, when used for information-gathering without digital interpersonal 'conversation', social media is a good thing. There is evidence for cyberbullying and the formation of adverse digital relationships with potential risks to self in the real world if a meeting is arranged with a deviant person. Finally, some social media uses can be viewed as potentially addictive; these can include preoccupations with gaming, especially when others are involved. Currently, therefore, young people themselves see good and bad things in social media [8, 9].

From the practitioner perspective, exploring and understanding the YP's social media life and determining if their current use is contributing to the presence of mental health problems are essential. Therapists should show an interest in how social media is used by the YP and discriminate between personal information-gathering and interpersonal connectivity use. If the latter is prevalent then consider the frequency, quality and impact that any 'chat' may be having. For some, this may be a negative connection to an unknown other or group and this will need to be reviewed and, where possible, reduced or stopped. If safeguarding the YP is needed then attend to the safeguarding and 'keeping you safe' rules discussed in Chapter 7. For some, however, social media use could be a strategy for improving mental health: this could include information-gathering. It could also include social connectivity that is planned and collaboratively agreed with the therapist for the purposes of improving prosocial networks, enhancing personal skills and/or educative gains. This can altogether be seen as enhancing well-being in the mentally unwell.

We are at the beginning of the era of digital tools in therapy and we can expect a substantial rise in their use soon. Currently, there is early evidence that digital therapy is effective with young people suffering from mild to moderate depression related health problems. We consider it unlikely that digital media will fully replace human therapists but hybrid interventions with both being used in brief therapies is very likely [10]. Indeed, there is every likelihood that digital information will be used as a support to psychological treatment strategies.

Here are some principles for assessing and evaluating digital lives and social media contributions to mental health:

- Digital and online resources can play an important role in supplementing face-to-face therapy and offering support in a way that is accessible to the YP.
- It is important to understand what types of digital/online tools they use and why. Aim to help the adolescent to use technology in an intentional, positive manner.
- It is essential to ask about these uses and digital lives to best understand the YP and formulate your therapeutic goals together whilst also ensuring they stay safe and supported.

Why Is Physical Activity Important?

Despite an enormous amount of interest in physical fitness, the relationship between physical and mental well-being in young people is not at all clear. Mentally unwell adolescents, however, are on average more sedentary than their mentally well counterparts and this may impact well-being by reducing educational progress and be associated with mental health problems [11].

Currently, we recommend that physical activity and exercise programmes designed to increase the level of activity in sedentary young people with mental health problems should be considered. We believe these should be made to be attractive and achievable for young people, emphasising the importance of a working collaborative approach to developing the activity. Activity should be tuned into obtaining regular, frequent activity spells that are likely to raise heart and breathing rates for ten minutes or more. This allows therapists to collaboratively fashion activity programmes that can be gentle and graded, with achievable goals for most adolescents.

Two physical activity principles for BPI:

- Physical activities can provide opportunities for positive reinforcement:
  o especially if linked to an individual's personal priorities around health, fitness, or weight
  o as well as social interaction
  o and a beneficial effect on self-esteem and sense of agency.
- Physical activity may be an adaptive distraction technique to reduce rumination and worry.

Work between Sessions for the Therapist and Others

In BPI there is an expectation that the therapist will offer some input between sessions to facilitate the YP's recovery, in the same way the YP is expected to. This is important to emphasise the collaborative nature of BPI. Between-session therapist input needs to be balanced with the importance of the adolescent's autonomy, with support from adults around them. Young people with more severe depression symptoms may require a greater degree of support from others at the beginning of therapy, which can be tailed off as their symptoms and functioning improve. Examples of between-session work are given in Table 8.3.

Culture and Diversity

It is important to be mindful and respectful of possible differences expressed in:

- race/ethnicity
- age
- culture
- sexuality
- disability
- gender
- spirituality.

Table 8.3 Between-session work examples

Example of therapist between-session work	Example of parent/carer between-session work
Phone call to family to update and explain the homework task	Meeting with school/college to discuss the best ways to support the YP
Contact with school/college to encourage support for the YP	Researching local clubs/resources to support an activity (e.g. finding out where the nearest rock-climbing wall is)
Exploring an app that the YP uses to consider how it could be helpfully used in therapy	Making changes to the YP's bedroom to facilitate good sleep (e.g. buying new curtains)
Learning more about a YP's interest/hobby to consider ideas for activities around this	Taking the YP food shopping and discussing food choices
Planning activities to complete during the next session	Spending time with the YP doing a physical activity or making food together or sharing a hobby/interest

Be aware that diversity is not always visible, so you need to be inclusive to invite opportunities for the YP to share information (e.g. not limiting relationship queries to heterosexual romantic partners). Refer to your training on diversity and inclusion for further guidance and take queries to supervision.

Endings in Therapy

As a likely source of stable positive reinforcement, the therapist should expect that the end of therapy may be challenging for a YP as this source of reinforcement will be lost. To help young people understand the brief nature of the work and encourage them to aim for independent progress after sessions end, the therapist should agree on the number of sessions at their first appointment and review this regularly throughout (e.g. 'Today is session three of six, so we'll have three more treatment sessions after today'). It is also important to make this clear to all involved in the care of the YP so there are realistic expectations. The therapist should be developing the ending plan *from the beginning of therapy*. Too often, the ending emerges without a plan and with no clear objective. We consider unplanned endings as therapeutically unwise and urge therapists to create a 'planned ending scenario' with clear objectives. This, of course, is a collaborative exercise with the YP.

- Clarify the tailing-off nature of the final sessions: bigger gaps between appointments towards the end will help the YP to try out making progress independently.
- Emphasise the expectation that progress will continue after sessions end, as new strategies take time to become familiar and impact on mood and functioning.
- Explicitly discuss who can help support the YP's progress once sessions end and how this will be put in place (e.g. a regular catch-up with mum to check in, meeting with a tutor once a week, etc.).
- Be mindful that young people who lack supportive adults in their life and/ or who have experienced the loss of important sources of positive reinforcement previously may find the ending of therapy particularly hard. Bring such cases to supervision.

REFERENCES

1. Orchard F, Gregory AM, Gradisar M, Reynolds S. Self-reported sleep patterns and quality amongst adolescents: cross-sectional and prospective associations with anxiety and depression. *J Child Psychol Psychiatry*. 2020;61(10):1126–37.
2. Orchard F, Pass L, Marshall T, Reynolds S. Clinical characteristics of adolescents referred for treatment of depressive disorders. *Child Adolesc Ment Health*. 2017;22(2):61–8.
3. Reynolds S, Orchard F, Midgley N, Kelvin R, Goodyer I, IMPACT consortium. Do sleep disturbances in depressed adolescents improve following psychological treatment for depression? *J Affect Disord*. 2020;262:205–10.
4. Force USPST, Krist AH, Davidson KW, Mangione CM, Barry MJ, Cabana M et al. Primary care-based interventions to prevent illicit drug use in children, adolescents, and young adults: US Preventive Services Task Force recommendation statement. *JAMA*. 2020;323(20):2060–6.
5. Houtepen LC, Heron J, Suderman MJ, Fraser A, Chittleborough CR, Howe LD. Associations of adverse childhood experiences with educational attainment and adolescent health and the role of family and socioeconomic factors: a prospective cohort study in the UK. *PLoS Med*. 2020;17(3):e1003031.
6. Erskine HE, Moffitt TE, Copeland WE, Costello EJ, Ferrari AJ, Patton G et al. A heavy burden on young minds: the global burden of

mental and substance use disorders in children and youth. *Psychol Med.* 2015;45(7):1551–63.

7. Kelly Y, Zilanawala A, Booker C, Sacker A. Social media use and adolescent mental health: findings from the UK Millennium Cohort Study. *EClinicalMedicine.* 2018;6:59–68.

8. O'Reilly M. Social media and adolescent mental health: the good, the bad and the ugly. *J Ment Health.* 2020;29(2):200–6.

9. O'Reilly M, Dogra N, Hughes J, Reilly P, George R, Whiteman N. Potential of social media in promoting mental health in adolescents. *Health Promot Int.* 2019;34(5):981–91.

10. Schleider JL, Mullarkey MC, Fox KR, Dobias ML, Shroff A, Hart EA, Roulston C. A randomized trial of online single-session interventions for adolescent depression during COVID-19. *Nat Hum Behav.* 2022;6(2):258–68.

11. Rodriguez-Ayllon M, Cadenas-Sanchez C, Estevez-Lopez F, Munoz NE, Mora-Gonzalez J, Migueles JH et al. Role of physical activity and sedentary behavior in the mental health of preschoolers, children and adolescents: a systematic review and meta-analysis. *Sports Med.* 2019;49(9):1383–410.

9 Top Tips for Best Practice

Here we provide our top tips for best practice. They are derived from clinical experiences and frequently asked questions during teaching and training of BPI.

Red Flags: Issues That Should Be Taken to Supervision

We have noted that, in our view, when undertaking any psychotherapy there should be supervision and reflective practice throughout one's career. Senior therapists can be as much in need of discussions about their cases as newly qualified practitioners. Until we have much improved our understanding of what intervention works for which patient and how, we recommend supervision as a key clinical tool in learning the skills and techniques of BPI. Of course, we do not yet know which of these tips is responsible for clinical effectiveness. Therefore, regular fortnightly supervision with a senior, more experienced colleague is sound practice. Table 9.1 describes key general components that should activate a discussion with your supervisor.

Table 9.1 Tips for taking queries to supervision

Issue	Why this should be taken to supervision
New case	To consider any challenges/opportunities present for this case at the start of the work; to ensure the supervisor is aware they are on your caseload.
Any risk identified	To support the therapist in managing this, consider risk management plan and whether additional input is required.
The YP or parent/carer is evasive when discussing risk information	May indicate a greater level of risk than is being disclosed; limited engagement in risk discussions may constitute increased risk (e.g. the safety plan not being implemented).

Table 9.1 (cont.)

Issue	Why this should be taken to supervision
Any indication the YP may not be willing to share risk information with parents/carers	Need to consider the balance of information-sharing vs therapeutic relationship when deciding on whether to break confidentiality without the YP's consent. (NOTE: this should be discussed immediately if there is a known risk and the YP does not consent to share. Seek immediate guidance from your supervisor.)
Drugs/alcohol/substance misuse	May need specialist input and that is a decision to be taken jointly with others.
Behaviour that is disorganised, suspicious, chaotic, out of the ordinary social withdrawal or otherwise strange	May indicate substance misuse, psychotic symptoms and/or neurological issues.
Non-attendance	Need for more assertive outreach; may indicate difficulties in forming a therapeutic alliance which need addressing.
Hostility/conflict between the YP and parents/carers in session	Need to address this for sessions to remain therapeutic and to maintain engagement; may need to have separate sessions with adults.
Any digital/online activity which you are not confident is safe or supervised appropriately	May indicate grooming/radicalisation or exposure to age-inappropriate material.
The YP mentions relationships with older individuals, without clear indication that family is aware and carefully monitoring this	May indicate power imbalance, exposure to age-inappropriate experiences and potentially exploitation/abuse that may not be legal and requires safeguarding action.
No treatment response after three sessions or observable rapid deterioration	May indicate poor engagement with treatment, difficulties in the therapeutic relationship or external factors that need addressing for the YP to make progress.
Physical health condition or physical health-related medication issues	May need to signpost to additional input (e.g. speak to GP/child health/paediatrics) or need to adapt therapy to take these factors into account. There may be a relationship between the physical health condition and current mental health; this should be considered. When the direction of

Table 9.1 (cont.)

Issue	Why this should be taken to supervision
	any effect is difficult to ascertain, seek additional medical advice (e.g. medication leading to drowsiness in the morning, unable to engage in some activities, a known physical condition that is not controlled and can have effects on mental well-being).
Impacts of any medication being prescribed for mental health	You should consider possible effects and side effects and discuss them carefully with your team medical prescriber/psychiatrist.
Need arising for medication for mental health	Remember that sometimes there is a role for psychotropic medication alongside talking therapies. Some young people come requesting this; take their requests seriously and consider pros and cons, and indications for and against carefully, in keeping with good practice guidelines (NICE). Discuss in supervision and with your team psychiatrist.
Any diversity issues that are identified	There may be issues relating to culture, spirituality, race/ethnicity, disability, gender, sexuality and other diversity issues that are important to consider in therapy. Supervision provides a space to consider these and whether therapy may need to be adapted (e.g. a teenage boy may find it difficult to share his emotions with a young female therapist; in some religions and cultures suicidal ideation is completely taboo and will not be discussed; a clash between the YP's sexuality and their parents'/carers' views may be an underlying conflict between them).

BPI Therapist Frequently Asked Questions (FAQs)

This final section describes the FAQs for the BPI therapist. Here we outline the day-to-day working realities (pragmatics) of BPI therapist behaviour. This provides a simple commentary on some key rules and parameters of clinical practice.

Table 9.2 Therapist role behaviours

What are the professional role behaviours of a BPI therapist?

- You are a coach, trainer, guide and collaborator who has expertise to share, not an 'expert' telling the YP what to do.
- You are there to provide guidance on mental illness, recovery and well-being through BPI. The adolescent is an expert on themselves and parents/carers/other adults in their life have important contributions that need hearing and evaluating.
- You must be mindful of your own actions in sessions: be positive in outlook, including thanking young people for their attendance at sessions and recognising their effort with BPI work (even if this is small or not as much as expected). Adopt the same approach with parents/carers and encourage them to do the same.
- You must be flexible: young people may respond differently to the tools and styles you can use and it's important to adapt to their needs.

Table 9.3 Collaboration

What does it mean to be collaborative?

- Collaboration = *the action of working with someone to effect a product.*
- It's a joint effort: there should be opportunities for all parties to contribute if needs dictate.
- This can be a challenge as many young people see adults in an authority-hierarchical role, so you need to work hard to help them understand that parents, siblings and others (teachers) may have a contribution to make that can improve clinical effectiveness and well-being.
- Parents also often view therapists as the 'expert': therapists should be authoritative but not authoritarian. Parents should get the idea of 'teamwork': the BPI therapist, the YP, their parents and perhaps other family members likely have different styles with differing perspectives but together they are 'greater than the sum of their parts' and can make a good team.
- Some simple steps can help:
  - Ask the YP what they would like to talk about in each session (and add it to a shared and explicit 'agenda' for the session).
  - 'Check in' with them before moving on from one topic to another.
  - Ask how each BPI topic relates to them.
  - Ask them for ideas for between-session work.
  - Use the Session Rating Scales/ROMs as a prompt for discussing your teamwork and how you need feedback from them to improve.
  - Empower them to be actively involved: they have control over the work; it's their life.

Table 9.4 Duration and timing of BPI

How should the sessions be spaced out?

- We recommend that, if possible, the first four sessions are completed within four to six weeks and subsequent sessions can take place every two to four weeks, depending on momentum and progress. This is so the young person can get started with making changes early on in treatment. Recall that rapid progress is made early and more sessions in the first few weeks can, we believe, enhance this rate of recovery.
- Check on holiday and other likely non-attendance dates at session 1 and plan around these. Check attendance dates with parents too.
- It's often helpful to signal endings at the beginning and to increase the gap between sessions towards the end of therapy. This helps to give the YP chance to make progress independently and prepare for ending. Indeed, note that we recommend planning for endings *soon after you begin* treatment.

Table 9.5 Activity log

How do I introduce an activity log in a way that feels acceptable to the YP?

- Introduce it to get to know them better, by learning about what they do every day.
- Be flexible. Work to their strengths (e.g. computer skills, use of mobile-based calendar/task lists).
- Be open about the need for this to work for *them* and agree a level of detail that is realistic. For some, the log is not feasible at all; others will very much like keeping a note of activities between sessions.

Table 9.6 Cognitive work

What should I do if the YP identifies thoughts in a certain situation? Is cognitive work part of BPI?

- BPI does not include any 'formal cognitive restructuring work' but it's important to validate the YP's experience and use that to better understand them.
- Help the YP to label the thought and identify how it made them feel.
- Help them focus on actions and behaviours by asking what the YP did in the situation and/or whether they would do anything differently next time.

Table 9.7 Self-harm and suicidality

How do I review and respond to a disclosure of self-harm or suicidal thoughts?

- **First of all, stick to your service's usual governance guidelines for managing safe-guarding and risk to self or others; BPI should fit seamlessly into usual practice.**
- **None of what follows should be taken as superseding your local service guidance or protocols.**
- Ask the YP about risk. For some this can be done with the parent/carer present; for others it needs to be with the parent/carer not present.
- In all cases re-check your clinical findings in case there is more information pertinent to these issues than you first considered.
- Check whether the YP would feel able to disclose this information and find a way to make this easier for them – for example, the therapist adding a question about self-harm to the end of the Revised Children's Anxiety and Depression Scale (RCADS).
- Normalise that self-harming and suicidal thoughts occur in some young people with mood-related mental illnesses. Explain that these thoughts often reduce as mood and depression improve. Check they have followed and understood this piece of psychoeducation.
- Ask the YP for details of the frequency and severity of the self-harm or suicidal thoughts so that you can monitor this and share information with the parent if necessary.
- Monitor and evaluate these thoughts and undertake safety checks every session. In BPI treatment responders there should be at least two further sessions where these are no longer reported. See below for guidelines for treatment non-responders.
- Take to supervision.

Table 9.8 Managing clinical content

How do I fit in all the other BPI content, if I have to have lots of risk discussions?

- It's fine to add one to two extra sessions if you need to take significant time to cover risk management.
- Be mindful that discussing risk and labelling the level of risk do not reduce risk; active steps need to be taken to manage and help to modify the risk and 'problems'.
- Remember that putting the BPI content into practice may improve the YP's mental health and reduce risk so it's important to cover this.
- Make any changes due to risk management clear to the family so they understand what is expected and why additional sessions may be required.
- Take to supervision.

Table 9.9 Low compliance with activity monitoring

What do I do if the YP has not completed their activity log?

- Do not tell them off or act like you are disappointed. It's better to suggest that you had not set this up well enough or indeed that it may not be a good fit for them.
- They may prefer to tell you than to keep a written record and that is fine too.
- If appropriate, identify barriers to completing the activity log, such as lack of explanation from yourself or overly high expectations of detail.
- Use problem-solving to identify what the YP could do to overcome these barriers.
- Emphasise that the YP can be creative in how they complete the activity log e.g. if the table does not appeal to them.
- Give praise for *any* attempts at completing the activity log.

Table 9.10 Ideas, activity and understanding

What are the most important ideas to get across with written and/or self-reported activity monitoring?

- There is a link between what you do, how you spend time and who with, and how you feel.
- There is no real 'no activity': you are always doing something and this can be open to change.
- The simplest things can make the biggest difference: noticing what you're doing and making small changes can have a big impact on your well-being.
- It is important to do things that matter to *you*, not just others.
- Do reinforce that considering doing activities and/or using an activity log is a way for the therapist to get to know the YP better.
- It doesn't matter how it's recorded, or indeed whether it's recorded or just remembered and discussed, as long as they can bring some information to sessions.

Table 9.11 Setting the difficulty bar just right

What if the young person struggles with reading and the workbook content is too difficult?

- Make this accessible so it works for them: edit the workbook-worksheets to include only the key points; check if they prefer diagrams/pictures.
- Consider audiotapes of the workbook-worksheets/sessions, if you have agreed the confidentiality of these.
- Use colour coding and symbols rather than words and numbers, e.g. ticks in green for enjoyment and a plus sign if it's an important activity to them.

Table 9.12 Young person in a hurry

What if a YP is keen to make changes from session 1?

- This is great, if they've understood the BPI rationale of changing behaviour in line with what's important to them and this fits with how they want to move forwards.
- They might already have some ideas of how they want to be with others and/or spend their time differently.
- Be clear that this is ok: encourage and support this and praise their motivation.
- Ask them to try to remember or record this in some way and make sure you discuss it in the next session (e.g. Which activities did you try to do more/less of? How did that affect your mood?).

Table 9.13 Keep it simple; do it well

Is BPI too simple to use with a complex case?

- BPI is as effective as CBT for complex depression cases. There is no clinical argument for a BPI therapist not to treat severe comorbid depressive illnesses.
- There is also evidence that the individual elements of BPI improve mental health (e.g. social prescribing and habilitation, psychoeducation, exercise, sleep, balanced diet, increasing meaningful activities).
- BPI can be used alongside additional interventions if clinically required: it is helpful if any other professional involved has a clear understanding of the ongoing BPI work.
- Use routine outcome measures (ROMs) and elicit client feedback regularly (e.g. every two weeks or every two sessions). This allows consideration of progress and can be used to prompt multidisciplinary team (MDT) discussions of whether an alternative approach may be more helpful if no progress is being made.

Table 9.14 Who is BPI for?

Might young people hear it as the therapist asking them to just 'do more'?

- That's not the message of BPI! Be very clear from the start that it's not just doing more. It's learning more about yourself and your mind, what helps and what doesn't. This includes, but is not limited to, doing more of *what matters to you* (not other people).
- Recall that seemingly simple changes can make big differences to mental health.
- Provide lots of careful listening, empathy and validation of their experience.
- This should include acknowledging the very real attempts made by the adolescent to change, now and in the past.
- Be clear with parents so they don't inadvertently find themselves providing an unhelpful message at home.

Table 9.15 Harmful risks from activity

What if a YP wants to engage in an activity I feel is harmful?

- This happens less often than you would expect, especially if you focus collaboratively on 'what matters' to the YP.
- If they do suggest an activity you find difficult to encourage (e.g. drug-taking), try to discuss the reasons and/or meaning behind the activity and brainstorm alternative activities that still fit (e.g. what matters = spending time with friends, activity = go to the skatepark together).
- Consider how these activities might be contrary to other things they hold as important (e.g. looking after myself).
- Provide psychoeducation (e.g. the negative impact drugs have on mental health).
- Bring this to supervision to discuss sharing information with parents/professionals.

Table 9.16 You hear what you want to hear

Won't a YP just tell me what matters/activities they think I want to hear?

- This is less common than you think if you have set up the collaboration-therapeutic relationship well!
- Some generic things that matter to the YP (e.g. doing well at school, being a good friend) are likely to apply to many young people, and activities can be individualised so it feels meaningful to the YP you're working with.
- The assessment details, content of early sessions and any verbal or written activity logging will give you both clearer ideas about the things that matter for the YP – highlighting these may encourage them to think more personally.

Table 9.17 Can BPI be enjoyable?

What if a YP engages in an activity but doesn't enjoy it?

- This is a possibility, especially in the early stages of treatment, so normalise this experience – enjoyment might take a little longer to come back or it may be the wrong activity for them now.
- Explore how the YP approached the activity. Were they fully engaged, e.g. they went out with friends but spent the whole time on their phone not speaking?
- If so, encourage them to engage fully with the activity, e.g. 'Next time you go out with friends, leave your phone in your pocket and join in the conversation!'
- Discuss how important the activity is – does it really matter to the young person? If not, identify another activity.

Table 9.17 (cont.)

What if a YP engages in an activity but doesn't enjoy it?

- If it does fit with what matters to them, reflect on and compare how the YP was experiencing activities before with how they are experiencing them now.
- Did they use to enjoy it before they were depressed?
- Discuss how some activities might be important and matter to them but not be enjoyable and, if neglected, lead to stress and problems (e.g. going for regular blood tests to keep a health condition monitored, in line with staying healthy).
- Some activities are not enjoyable in the short term but lead to positive reinforcement over a longer period (e.g. exercise may not be fun now but feeling like you're getting fitter is good for well-being once it starts to get easier).

Table 9.18 Disagreement between parents and young person about activity choices

What if the YP identifies an activity their parents/carers don't agree with?

- This could happen if a parent has different things that matter to their child. Be clear with parents about the rationale for doing personally important activities (to gain a sense of reward from life) and discuss why this activity is important to the YP.
- Negotiate the activity – are there any compromises that can be reached?
- Use contracts or problem-solving within session to facilitate discussion and compromise.
- Remember, your primary aim is to support the YP to implement what matters to them, and sometimes finding ways of negotiating that with parents/carers turns out to be part of the treatment, helping the young person and family communicate differently.

Table 9.19 Specific, clear and meaningful

How should I make goals SMART and BPI-specific?

- Try to make goals as specific as possible. If the YP identifies a feeling for their goal such as 'To feel less down', try asking, 'How would you know you were feeling that way?' and 'What would you be doing that you are not doing now?'
- Look at the 'Making sense of things' section (especially 'What do I hope to change?') for possible goals.
- Agree a time frame for when the YP wants to achieve their goal.
- Use specific examples to agree what certain numbers on the goals progress chart would look like to them – what would they be doing in order to rate a 5/10 or 10/10?

Table 9.20 Routine measures and their meaning

How do I use the questionnaires (ROMs) in a clinically meaningful way?

- Make sure you understand the ROMs yourself and are familiar with individual items so you can use this data meaningfully.
- Score these up as soon as possible: for example, the RCADS depression subscale can be quickly summed in session; the Outcome Rating Scale (ORS)/Session Rating Scale (SRS) can be 'eyeballed' in session (and measured afterwards). You can ask the YP to help score these in session, and the full RCADS can be calculated and graphs printed after session.
- Make use of any computer programs you have access to that enable scoring in session.
- Plot the RCADS depression subscale and ORS on a graph across sessions (manually or on a computer program), using different lines for the YP and parent reports, and consider how to share these with the YP and parent/carer during sessions.
- Include clinical thresholds for both YP and parent scores.
- *Always* discuss ROMs with the young person and if possible their parent/carer if you have asked for them to be completed.
- Plot the SRS across sessions: see if there is anything (big or small) that the YP would like to do differently.
- Ask the YP and parent for feedback on what they think the scores are suggesting and if they are a true reflection of how they are doing.
- Be clear about how gathering this information adds to the other sources of information – they all matter, not just the ROMs (e.g. verbal report, therapist view).
- Discuss ROMs in supervision.

Table 9.21 The BPI therapist is stuck

Help! I feel like I am stuck with a BPI client – what do I do?

- Use supervision to discuss your concerns: what makes you feel 'stuck'?
- Ask the YP for feedback. How are they finding the sessions? What do they think you could do differently that might help?
- Think about BPI topics that might help: reformulating, problem-solving, focusing on healthy habits or involving others.
- Have you covered all the BPI menu items and, if so, what is the current formulation? Remember the formulation is pivotal and if there is no progress, chances are you have missed something in the formulation.
- Consider external (e.g. bullying, traumatic events or practical matters like lack of transport) and internal (fatigue, irritability, hopelessness) barriers to change for the YP.

Table 9.21 (cont.)

Help! I feel like I am stuck with a BPI client – what do I do?

- Use the ORS and SRS and review or listen back to your therapy sessions to look for clues about what might be stopping progress. Consider this in the light of your formulation.
- Consider whether your own and the client's expectations are realistic: progress might be being made, just at a slower rate than hoped for.
- The 'emotional contagion' aspect of depression can impact on therapists' sense of optimism and change – remember this and reorient your own approach accordingly.

Table 9.22 Ending BPI

How do I manage the ending of BPI?

- Consensual agreement about ending is important.
- *Plan BPI in six-session blocks with the caveat that there can be an agreed ending during that time or at the planned end.*
- Refer to the planned ending throughout your work. (e.g. 'today is session four of six', 'we have two sessions left together').
- Be aware that you may be a source of positive reinforcement for the YP and that ending sessions may remove this. It is important to find other ways to get this reinforcement from their everyday relationships, family, friends and/or the wider environment, school/college, etc.
- Some people may find endings harder than others: young people who have experienced interpersonal losses or traumas and those who have established a strong therapeutic relationship with you may find this more difficult.
- Parents/carers often worry about sessions ending, so be clear about how they can get support after your sessions end. Signpost to the resources in the workbook. Enlist their support to keep things going after therapy has finished.
- Be realistic: use the learning from their workbook to discuss potential setbacks and how they can use their new skills to overcome these.
- Reinforce that the changes that have been made are due to their hard work and be optimistic and positive that they can continue to do this after sessions have finished.
- *Before* the final session, ask how the YP would like to say goodbye at the review (e.g. shake hands, hug, say goodbye).

Table 9.23 Extending BPI

Can I offer any top-up sessions after the review?

- Discuss in supervision: sometimes it is not always helpful to keep offering sessions and discharge can be a positive experience for the YP to feel they have control over their own mental health.
- BPI top-up sessions could be used if the YP started to feel low again following treatment – if they are still in the service.
- If six sessions are deemed with your supervisor to be insufficient to reduce illness and improve well-being, then prescribe another six. You can then replan ending with the young person within these next six sessions.
- Recall that research trials data from real-life clinical settings shows that around 50% of responders need around 6 sessions or fewer; a further 45% will need 7 to 12 sessions and the last 5% of likely responders may need 13 to 18 sessions.
- Troubleshooting can be used for anything that has prevented progress. Validate the normality of setbacks and refer to their end-of-treatment relapse prevention plan.
- One in five of all cases, across any psychotherapy treatment, are likely to not respond. Currently, however, we cannot predict from assessment who the non-responders are likely to be. So consider a flattening progress curve (symptoms and impairment) after 6 to 12 sessions. These cases must be discussed with your supervisor as early as possible in the 'non-response mode'.

Table 9.24 Information and support

Where can I go to get more information on BPI?

- Your supervisor.
- Colleagues who are also delivering BPI: it can really help to hear about other cases.

Index

For EU product safety concerns, contact us at Calle de José Abascal, 56–1°, 28003 Madrid, Spain or eugpsr@cambridge.org.

www.ingramcontent.com/pod-product-compliance
Ingram Content Group UK Ltd.
Pitfield, Milton Keynes, MK11 3LW, UK
UKHW040946090126
466816UK00019B/297